RCGP Handbook of Sexual Health in Primary Care

Yvonne Carter
Catti Moss
Anne Weyman
Editors

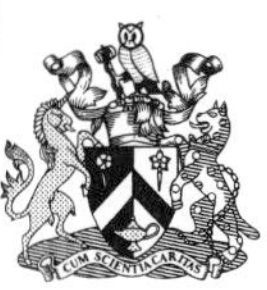

produced in collaboration with the Family Planning Association

FPA
FAMILY PLANNING
ASSOCIATION

The Royal College of General Practitioners was founded in 1952, with this object:

'To encourage, foster and maintain the highest possible standards in general medical practice and for that purpose to take or join with others in taking steps consistent with the charitable nature of that object which may assist towards the same.'

Among its responsibilities under its Royal Charter, the College is entitled to:

'Diffuse information on all matters affecting general medical practice and issue such publications as may assist the object of the College.'

Published by the Royal College of General Practitioners, 14 Princes Gate, London SW7 1PU

Designed and typeset by Andrew Haig & Associates
Printed in Great Britain by the College Hill Press Limited

ISBN 0 85084 238 7

contents

acknowledgements

We would like to thank all those who have made this book possible. The Margaret Pyke Memorial Trust and the Royal College of General Practitioners (RCGP) have generously contributed the production costs. The Family Planning Association (FPA) has contributed with writers and editors. In particular we would like to thank Toni Belfield of the FPA for her valuable comments and advice. Our thanks also go to Jane Hobden, freelance editor, who polished the text and took the book through its various production stages. The RCGP has provided the inspiration, secretarial backup, authors' travel expenses, and the majority of the authors and editors. The authors have worked incredibly hard, with very tight schedules, and impossible deadlines. Our heartfelt thanks go to everyone involved in this project. We give particular praise to the outstanding efforts of Fiona van Zwanenberg without whose help the book would never have gone to press.

The RCGP Sexual Health Task Group acknowledges, with thanks, the support of the Margaret Pyke Memorial Trust in producing this handbook

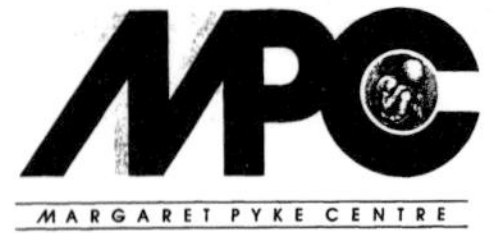

Table of abbreviations

AIDS – acquired immune deficiency syndrome
BV – bacterial vaginosis
COC – combined oral contraceptive
D&C – dilatation and curettage
DMPA – depot medroxyprogesterone acetate
hCG – human chorionic gonadotrophin
HIV – human immunodeficiency virus
HPV – human papilloma virus
HSV – herpes simplex virus
IUD – intrauterine device
IUS – intrauterine system
LAM – lactational amenorrhoea method
NSGI – non-specific genital infection
NSU – non-specific urethritis
PCC – postcoital contraception
PID – pelvic inflammatory disease
POP – progestogen only pill
PSA – prostate specific antigen
STI – sexually transmitted infection
TOP – termination of pregnancy
UTI – urinary tract infection
VTE – venous thromboembolism

foreword

Fulfilling and healthy sexual relationships enhance people's vitality and can nurture good relationships. But sexual activity can have undesirable consequences as well, such as unplanned pregnancy, emotional problems, infection and infertility. It is also an area where embarrassment and misinformation are common. Where better to address such issues than in family medical practice where most aspects of care and the fostering of good health occur.

This book, produced in response to requests from primary care teams, provides a rich source of evidence-based recommendations across the spectrum of sexual health. It is particularly pleasing to see issues addressed such as access, appropriate identification and management of problems, multi-disciplinary working, and quality; in addition to topics such as men's sexual health and preconception care.

I believe that all those in primary care will find the information in this handbook clear to understand and simple to incorporate into their everyday practice. For many of those seeking such advice in primary care this should lead to an indispensable improvement in their well-being. It will also be a significant contribution to an important area of public health.

Sir Kenneth Calman
Chief Medical Officer

> 'If sex is such a natural phenomenon, how come there are so many books on how to?'
> *Bette Midler*

preface

Yvonne Carter
Catti Moss
Anne Weyman

Sexual health is central to each individual's well-being. So it is hardly surprising that when the Royal College of General Practitioners (RCGP) asked members what issues they would like the College to address, sexual health topped the poll. This handbook, which is a collaborative venture between the RCGP and the Family Planning Association (FPA), aims to meet that need, both for health professionals working in general practice today and for students who plan to do so in the future.

The term 'sexual health' is not in general usage, nor is it easy to define. It can affect a person's physical, emotional, spiritual and mental well-being. It has been defined as 'the enjoyment of the sexual activity of one's choice without causing or suffering physical or mental harm'. The ability to make decisions about and take responsibility for sexual expression is influenced by social, economic, cultural and educational factors. Health professionals therefore need a wide range of skills to be effective in this area. As the following facts illustrate, it is a vital one for general practice:

- A fifth of pregnancies end in abortion
- A third of live births are unintended
- It is estimated that most women will have an unintended pregnancy at some stage in their reproductive life, and 40 per cent will have a termination
- There were 400,000 new cases of sexually transmitted infections in 1995
- up to 10 per cent of sexually active young people have chlamydia
- A sixth of couples seek assistance for infertility

These are worrying figures and reflect a great unmet need for professional skills and services.

The Health of the Nation document, published by the last Government in 1993, recognised the importance of sexual health and identified these key objectives:

- to reduce the incidence of HIV infection
- to reduce the incidence of sexually transmitted infections
- to reduce the number of unintended pregnancies

In translating these general objectives into specific targets, the emphasis was placed on reducing the incidence of gonorrhoea and the conception rate for under 16s. In fact, HIV/AIDS and teenage conceptions have been the main focus of activity. In general practice, our longitudinal relationship with patients and involvement with families and communities, make it clear that the problem areas are more widespread. General figures for sexually transmitted infections and terminations of pregnancy show the present scale of these problems.

Sexually transmitted infections in England in 1995

New cases seen at NHS genitourinary medicine clinics

Genital warts virus	93,317
Chlamydia	39,289
Herpes	27,065
Gonorrhoea	12,359
Trichomoniasis	5,486
Scabies	5,478
Syphilis	1,416

In addition there were 3,903 new cases of HIV/AIDS reported in 1995.

Department of Health, 1996

These figures do not include sexually transmitted infections that were treated in locations other than GUM clinics. In the case of infections like chlamydia, many sufferers are treated in general practice or gynaecology clinics. Many others, being symptom free, remain undetected, so the actual incidence will be much higher.

The stigma and ignorance associated with sexually transmitted infections make it difficult for patients to raise their concerns or to seek advice about symptoms. Although GUM clinics have excellent systems to protect confidentiality, patients may fear that just by attending a clinic they may risk being seen in the wrong part of the hospital. The fears about confidentiality are even greater in general practice, perhaps because it is much more familiar, and staff are less anonymous than in the hospital. There may be special fears if the partner is a patient in the same practice.

Most general practitioners and practice nurses have received little or no training in this area, either at undergraduate or professional level. We hope that this handbook will remedy this to the point where primary care workers can confidently start to tackle this epidemic, either alone or in association with their local GUM clinic.

The figures below demonstrate that the problem of unintended pregnancy does not just relate to teenagers. As women in their twenties are less likely to terminate an unplanned pregnancy, the numbers of these must be even greater. It is clear that women of all ages are not able to control their fertility in the way that they would wish.

Termination rates for residents of England and Wales in 1995

	rate per 1000	number
under 16	5.2	3,270
16–19	21.7	24,945
20–24	25.5	43,394
25–29	18.6	37,254
30–34	12.4	25,759
35–39	7.9	14,352
40–44	2.9	4,868

Although the number of women in the 40-44 age group who have terminations is very small, 40 per cent of conceptions in this age group end in abortion.

Abortion statistics 1995, Office for National Statistics, 1997

Traditionally, many women have used family planning clinics for their contraceptive care. Now in some areas, health authorities are focusing on providing services to the younger age group, and general practice is being relied upon on to fill the gap. It is essential that GPs and practice nurses are in a position to advise about the advantages and disadvantages of all the various methods so that the user can choose the one that will suit them best. Having chosen, the GP or nurse needs the skills to provide that method, or to arrange for someone else to do so.

Young people especially have enormous concerns about confidentiality when they receive contraception through general practice. Recent studies have shown that 75 per cent of patients who are under 16 are afraid that their GP cannot, or will not, maintain confidentiality regarding contraception. But this is not just a problem for the under 16s – all ages have concerns about general practice confidentiality, and it is a major barrier to the effective supply of services. The problem will not be solved easily, but great improvements can be made by both improving our practice in this area, and by publicising our policies on confidentiality.

Fears about confidentiality are not the only barriers to effective sexual health care in general practice. The variations in teaching sexual health in the undergraduate medical curriculum means that many doctors have difficulty taking a sexual history. They may be embarrassed talking about sex at all. Nurses too get little training in talking about sexual matters with patients. Patients, who may have had little or no sex education, need a skilled, unembarrassed, sympathetic approach to help them talk freely in this difficult area. Enquiries to the FPA helpline show that older women are frequently unwilling to ask questions of their doctors or nurses because they feel they should already have the necessary knowledge and are afraid of appearing foolish.

This handbook has been written by people from a wide range of backgrounds: general practice, nursing, family planning, obstetrics, genitourinary medicine, psychosexual medicine, audit, and academic departments. Sometimes we had difficulty with the terms to use, and had to choose between alternatives. We chose to use the abbreviation IUD rather than IUCD for intrauterine contraceptive devices, in line with WHO usage, and despite the potential confusion with intrauterine death. The debate was more heated about whether we would talk about sexually transmitted diseases or sexually transmitted infections. In the end we opted for STIs, as the author of that chapter preferred. We hope it will not confuse those who are used to talking about STDs. Another ongoing debate in the sexual health field is whether to use the term 'client' instead of 'patient'. In view of the primary care professionals for whom we are writing, we decided to use the term 'patient', while recognising that those seeking advice on contraceptive and sexual health are not, in most cases, being treated for an illness.

This book is intended as a practical guide to gaining basic skills in sexual health care. It is aimed at all those who provide these services in primary care whether nurses running well-woman or young people's clinics, or GPs in every day surgeries. We hope it will be especially useful for GP registrars, who often find that a spell in gynaecology does not prepare them for the range of problems in primary care. Undergraduate students will also find this book valuable, especially if they intend to go into general practice, urology, gynaecology, or a related area.

The editors have tried to cover all the relevant topics in the handbook. It has been designed to complement the *FPA contraceptive handbook*: both books will be included in the FPA's forthcoming contraceptive pack for primary care professionals – on which the RCGP is collaborating.

We will have succeeded in our aims if this handbook finds a place on the bookshelves of busy practitioners, to be referred to when guidance is needed on a particular issue, or to be browsed through at length. We hope that it will enable professionals to improve sexual health services in primary care, creating clinics and surgeries that are appropriate for their patients with a friendly and non-judgmental atmosphere. Above all, this handbook offers practical guidance on how to provide a high quality service to patients, so giving them access to the best possible standard of sexual health care.

September 1997

Yvonne Stedman

chapter one

accessibility of sexual health services

part

I

introduction

The Shorter Oxford Dictionary defines 'accessible' as 'capable of being entered or approached.' No matter how distinctive, modern and attractive the sexual health services' facilities are, if clients are not aware of them, able to approach and to use them then the facilities become inappropriate and a waste of resources.

Sexual health has been defined as: *'enjoyment of sexual activity of one's choice, without causing or suffering physical or mental harm'*[1].

This definition was adopted by a consensus workshop on sexual health promotion and service delivery in March 1995.

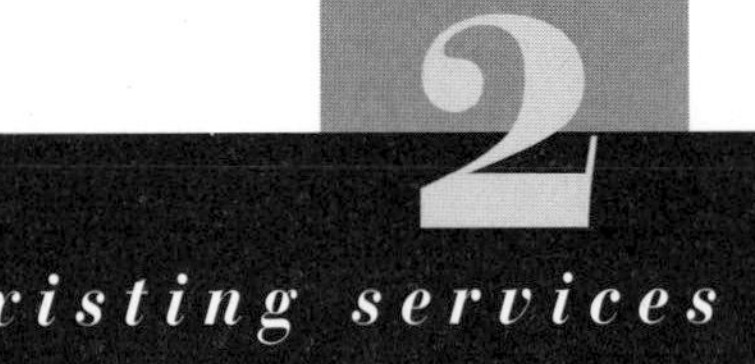

existing services

The components of sexual health care include those services involved in the prevention and management of sexually transmitted infections (STIs) and unintended pregnancies, the prevention of reproductive morbidity and the prevention of sexual dysfunction.

Existing sexual health services are provided through a variety of outlets, principally in general practice, family planning clinics and genitourinary medicine (GUM) clinics. For the sexual health care professional there is little national information on sexual health services in terms of:

- who does and who does not use particular services
- why services are or are not used
- where services are and how people access them
- whether existing services meet actual or perceived needs, or not

The limited research that is available is often small scale and population specific.

According to Ketting[1a], in an appraisal of contraception in Western Europe, the quality of family planning and contraceptive use depends, primarily, on three main factors:

- ample availability of contraceptives
- easily accessible and good quality services,
- sufficient knowledge of contraception and motivation for use

Since 1974 the availability of contraceptives has not been a problem in the UK. However, accessibility, knowledge and motivation are issues that are intrinsically linked and have still to be resolved successfully.

The reorganisation of the National Health Service (NHS) in 1974 allowed free family planning services in community clinics and hospitals. This was extended to include primary care in 1975. Some voluntary organisations such as the Brook Advisory Centres also provide free contraceptive services.

Government policy, as outlined by the Department of Health in 1990[2] makes it clear that people should have access to a choice of provider for family planning services by allowing dual provision through GPs, clinics in the community and in hospitals. In 1992 guidelines for reviewing services[3] were issued to regional health authorities in England. These gave advice on targeting and accessibility of services, information about services offered, sex education and the needs of the young. Current Department of Health guidance[4] stresses the importance of family planning as a health care service, and the need for close liaison between the different agencies at both provider and purchaser level, to ensure that the various family planning services are complementary. The balance of services needs to match local needs.

The Health of the Nation document[5] states that the development of GUM services and the establishment of easily accessible GUM provision for the residents of every health district should be a priority within the NHS. Attendance rates vary throughout the country, which in part reflect the incidence of STIs but also the accessibility and availability of services.

How accessible are existing services?
Providers should look at current services and determine whether or not they meet identified needs. While they should meet the needs of the 'general client group', it is also important to assess the take up of services by those whose current usage is lowest, but who, nevertheless, have an identifiable need.

A principal aim of any sexual health service must be to ensure that potential clients know of its existence. Whether it is contraceptive services within general practice, screening for infection within genito-urinary medicine, or sexual health education, the service must be accessible, attractive and appropriate to those men and women who need to use them.

The focus of existing services has often been to address sexual health problems rather than adopting a positive attitude towards promoting sexual health and to developing links with education. In some cases, the result has been a lack of information about the services on offer, long waits for appointments, unwelcoming reception staff and unattractive surroundings. Even for the confident, able-bodied adult with developed communication skills, accessing some services can be a formidable obstacle course. We should perhaps ask ourselves how much harder it is for young people, for people with physical or learning disabilities or for those whose first language is not English.

Amongst some providers of sexual health services, there may be the perception that certain groups are not sexually active or sexual activity may be disapproved of. Accessibility of services in these cases may therefore never have been seen as an issue.

The following groups may have particular difficulties accessing current services:

- young people, particularly young men
- people with disabilities such as:
  - chronic physical disease
  - physical disabilities
  - learning disabilities
  - chronic mental illness
- people from minority ethnic groups
- gay men, lesbians and bisexuals

part 3

identifying the need for sexual health services

Health authorities, commissioning departments, GPs, trusts, education providers, social services and the voluntary sector providing sexual health services must work together in order to evaluate and develop existing services to meet the needs of users and potential users of sexual health services and to identify unmet needs.

Useful sources of information on activity trends and people's needs for sexual health services include:

- Korner (KT31 and KC60) data and other local data on size of client groups and current use of services
- commissioning departments can identify GPs' item of service payments for contraceptive care
- ONS – regional data on births by women's age, marital status, pregnancy outcome and abortion statistics

part 4

what sexual health services does the practice /clinic provide?

Any GP or clinic providing sexual health services needs to assess their existing services to ensure accessibility and appropriateness:

- Are all methods of contraception available? Are patients aware if some methods are not available and where, under such circumstances, they can be found? For example, if a practitioner does not fit intrauterine devices (IUDs), are women informed of its availability from another provider?
- Is there a choice of female or male doctor? This is often an important factor for ethnic groups or young women
- How easy is it to access postcoital contraception (PCC)? This may provide a chance to give opportunistic sexual health advice and to discuss future contraception
- Do you provide 'on the spot' pregnancy testing? Again this is an opportunity to see the worried client who may have taken a risk
- Are you able to address other sexual health issues such as STI infection or psychosexual issues? Who do you refer to when faced with a problem beyond your experience or skills?
- Are special services provided for young people, ethnic groups, the disabled or other identifiable groups within the local community?

Appropriateness
Taking account of the social and demographic variation and the constraints of local geography, sexual health care professionals

need to ask how their services can be geared to meeting the local needs that have been identified.

Accessibility of provision

Where is the practice or clinic? Is it near to schools and colleges or town centres? Can the service be reached easily by public transport? Is there a choice of times? Is it an 'appointment only' or walk-in service?

Information and advertising

How are services advertised? Are family planning services mentioned separately in practice leaflets? How easy is it for patients to find information in local telephone directories about family planning and genitourinary medicine? Do clinics provide leaflets for distribution? Who should be involved in leaflet distribution and where should they be? What ethnic groups live in your service area and are leaflets available in the requisite languages?

Training and education

What training do staff have? Do the doctors hold the Joint Certificate on Contraception (JCC) or Diploma in Family Planning and Reproductive Health Care? Do the nurses hold their family planning qualification (ENB901)? Do staff have further training needs to address the wider issues of sexual health?

Links with other sexual health service providers

What links do you have with other providers? Is there a local forum for sexual health service providers to ensure the complimentary nature of services and to identify gaps in service provision?

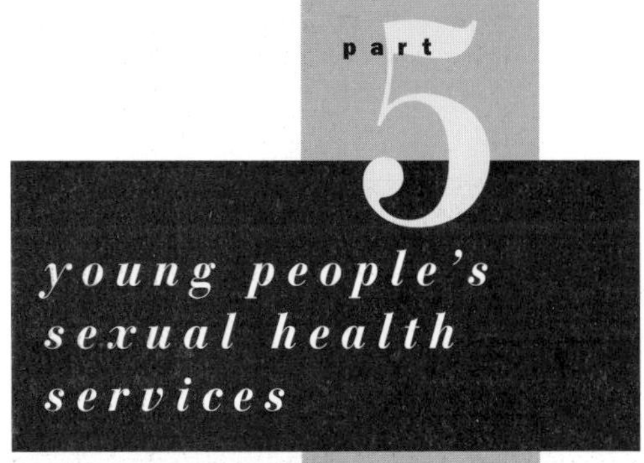

part 5 young people's sexual health services

The UK has the dubious distinction of having the highest teenage pregnancy rate among 15-19 year olds in Western Europe. While this rate has decreased from its all time high in 1990, it currently stands at 56.8 per 1000. A third of pregnancies among 16–19 year olds are terminated[6] and half of conceptions among those under 16 years of age end in termination. The personal, physical and psychological costs of these figures to the individuals concerned are incalculable, and the financial costs to the NHS are considerable. Teenage pregnancy is associated with increased risk of poor social, economic and health outcomes for both mother and child.

The *Effective Health Care*[7] bulletin on teenage pregnancy made media headlines following its publication in February 1997, when it summarised research evidence on approaches to preventing teenage pregnancy and on alleviating its direct negative health and social effects[8,9]. The document seeks to inform decisions made on the best ways of developing, organising, delivering and monitoring services to young people.

PREVENTING AND REDUCING THE ADVERSE EFFECTS OF UNINTENDED PREGNANCIES

Teenage pregnancy is associated with increased risk of poor social, economic and health outcomes for both mother and child

A factor strongly associated with deferring pregnancy is good general education

The health and development of teenage mothers and their children has been shown to benefit from programmes promoting access to antenatal care, targeted support by health visitors, social workers or 'lay mothers' and provision of social support, educational opportunities and pre-school education

School-based sex education can be effective in reducing teenage pregnancy especially when linked to access to contraceptive services. The most reliable evidence shows that it does not increase sexual activity or pregnancy rates

Contraceptives when used properly are highly cost effective and can result in significant savings

Increasing the availability of contraceptive clinic services for young people is associated with reduced pregnancy rates

Contraceptive services should be based on an assessment of local needs and ensure accessibility and confidentiality

Reproduced from *Effective Health Care, February 1997*

Is there a need for special provision?

The RCOG report on unplanned pregnancy in 1989[10], had previously highlighted the particular problems of teenage pregnancies. It recommended that special contraceptive clinics for teenagers be provided. The Health of the Nation strategy also identified the prevention of teenage pregnancies as a priority, with a target to reduce the rate of conceptions from 9.6 per 1000 in 1989 to 4.8 per 1000 by the year 2000. Current data suggests that this target is unlikely to be achieved.

Before 1975 very few under 16 year olds attended family planning clinics. Since then the proportion has risen steadily, apart from the effect caused by the Gillick case in the mid-1980s[11]. By 1995-96 an estimated 10 per cent of 14-15 year olds were attending clinics. In 1975, the proportion of 16–19 year olds attending clinics was 15 per cent and by 1995–96 this had risen to 19 per cent. As the Effective Health Care bulletin's review of recent economic evaluations shows[12,13] family planning services are highly cost effective and provide a high rate of return to the NHS. These economic calculations show that the costs of providing contraceptive services are far less than the health and social costs of unplanned pregnancies[14,15].

How will this service be provided?

The 1992 NHS guidelines[3] for reviewing family planning services, identified young people as a group who showed relatively poor uptake of contraceptive services. At the same time their need for separate, less formal, family planning arrangements was emphasised. Studies have shown an improvement in service use and decreased conception rates when services are provided by clinics or youth orientated clinics[16].

Two types of service are suggested by a report compiled by the Policy Studies Institute[17]: 'direct services' offering contraceptive services to young people at a defined base, and 'outreach services' to go out to young people or to support those working with young people.
Direct services should include clinics designated for young people within GP surgeries or community clinics offering:

- contraceptive advice and supplies
- emergency contraception
- infection screening
- pregnancy testing and counselling
- medical cover

The service could support satellite drop-in locations within youth centres offering sexual health advice and education, on the spot pregnancy testing and counselling.

Young men remain a difficult group to reach and the numbers which access existing services continue to be low. Contraceptive services are currently heavily female orientated and often have mainly female staff. It is important to have appropriately trained male staff within young people's clinics and to ensure that potential male users are aware of this fact. Boyfriends and girlfriends should be encouraged to take joint responsibility for their sexual health so make it clear that they can attend together.

Timing and location of clinics
Young people's clinics are more likely to attract young people if they are provided in the late afternoon, early evening or Saturday mornings and afternoons. Young people want 'easy to find' but not too public a service site. A town or city centre location is best, but not one on the high street.

Structure of the clinic
An informal and friendly atmosphere without too clinical an atmosphere is more likely to attract young people. Reception staff should be welcoming and non-judgmental in order to encourage continued attendance and to motivate clinic users to make recommendations to friends. Young people often find it helpful to be seen with a friend and staff need to be confident in offering 'group consultations'.

Young people need to be given clear, factual information in a straightforward, non-judgmental manner which allows them to make informed choices. Involvement of local school nurses in young people's clinics will often provide a vital link between the service and potential clients. To meet the different and often overlapping needs of young people there should be an appropriate skill mix amongst staff to include medical, counselling and educational expertise.

Confidentiality
Confidentiality and anonymity are common concerns of young people who often need reassurance on such matters. Having a confidentiality statement, such as the one below, displayed in the waiting area is often helpful.

CONFIDENTIALITY STATEMENT

This is a completely confidential service

Even if you are under 16, doctors and nurses still have to keep anything you tell them in private just as they would for an adult

---

We will not discuss any information about you with anyone else, unless you ask us to do so, except in very exceptional circumstances – if your or any other person' s safety is at risk

---

In these exceptional circumstances you will be kept fully informed

Initially the recording of information should be kept to a minimum and formal notes only made out if contraception other than barrier methods is going to be prescribed. Information should only be passed to the young person's GP with their expressed consent. Particular care should be taken over recording correspondence wishes such as whether letters can be sent to a home address.

Staff dealing with young people should be familiar with the Gillick guidelines given by Lord Fraser (sometimes known as the 'Fraser guidelines'):

GILLICK OR 'FRASER' GUIDELINES

A doctor or other professional would be justified in giving advice and treatment without parental knowledge or consent, provided he is satisfied:

- **that the young person could understand his advice and had sufficient maturity to understand what was involved in terms of the moral, social and emotional implications**
- **that he could neither persuade the young person to inform the parents, nor to allow him to inform them, that contraceptive advice was being sought**
- **that the young person would be very likely to begin, or to continue having, sexual intercourse with or without contraceptive treatment**
- **that, without contraceptive advice or treatment, the young person's physical or mental health would be likely to suffer**
- **that the young person's best interests required him to give contraceptive advice, treatment or both without parental consent**

The leaflet *Confidentiality and people under 16* contains guidance in dealing with this age group[18].

Promoting the service

Ideally advertising should be aimed at both young people themselves and professionals concerned with this age group. The planning of any new young person's service should involve local young people in order to ensure that the new services are appropriate and accessible. When the new clinic is launched, inform the local press and radio, and distribute posters, leaflets and cards in appropriate places such as youth clubs, schools, community centres, cafes, and bus and railway stations

Young people's services should be integrated with mainstream sexual health services. Liaison with other agencies concerned with young people is vital. Local multi-disciplinary advisory groups would ensure a strategic approach to the provision of young people's services.

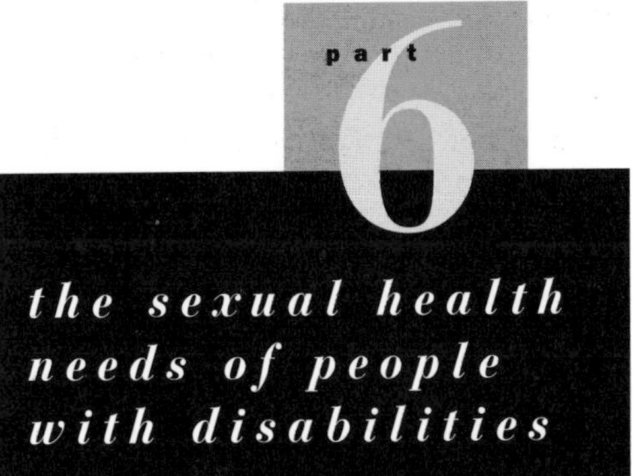

part 6 the sexual health needs of people with disabilities

As Cooper points out[19], clinicians need to remember that disabled patients are people first, disabled second. Disabled people have the same rights and expectations as 'non-disabled' people. This includes the right to fulfilling sexual relationships, although society often gives the message that disabled people should not be sexually active. Access to GP surgeries or family planning clinics may be difficult and disabled people may be unsure of their welcome[20] should they attend. How many clinics or surgeries have wheelchair access, have information leaflets in Braille or audiotapes? How easy would it be to examine a person in a wheelchair in the average clinic/surgery setting?

Other avenues for reaching visually impaired people may also need to be explored, such as advertising on local radio or informing local organisations.

Certain disabilities may directly affect a person's sexual health and their ability to access sexual health services. These include:

- people with chronic physical disease such as multiple sclerosis, diabetes or arthritis
- people with physical disabilities such as paraplegia which may be congenital or acquired
- people with learning difficulties who may also have physical disabilities
- people with chronic mental illness

Disabled young people will experience the same traumas of adolescence as their non-disabled peers but they may receive no or limited sex education within special schools which reduces their access to information and advice[21].

Professionals in primary care or clinics often have little or no training in dealing with sexuality and disability. Different skills and knowledge will be necessary to offer disabled patients the sexual health services they need. It may be helpful to liaise with colleagues who have experience in helping people with particular disabilities.

What services should be provided?

People with disabilities are likely to have a combination of sexual health needs which are emotional, physical and contraceptive[19]. Sexual dysfunction may be a particular problem for physically ill or handicapped people. In one study 50 per cent of middle aged men with insulin dependent diabetes reported erectile dysfunction[22]. Another study showed that between 50 per cent and 90 per cent of patients with multiple sclerosis develop sexual difficulties[23/24]. How often is a sexual history taken from a person with such chronic disabilities as diabetes or multiple sclerosis? All too often these needs are never identified and treated because the major effects of the disease are more prominent in the doctor's mind. There may also be a subconscious collusion between the patient and the doctor ensuring that the patient is reluctant to admit to sexual dysfunction in case of embarrassment or dismissal by the doctor. Further, the clinician may give little if any opportunity to the patient to introduce into the consultation any discussion of sexual dysfunction because of the clinician's own embarrassment and inadequacy at dealing with such problems.

Patients with complex medical and sexual needs are often deprived of an holistic approach. In 1987, Maurice[25], reported that the only way to help people with such diverse and complex sexual health is by adopting a multi-disciplinary approach. Joint clinics with input from gynaecologists, family planning doctors, urologists, psychosexual clinicians and psychiatrists might be the first step in developing an appropriate service for such patients.

A person's emotional and psychological needs may focus on issues such as self-esteem, and on coming to terms with their disability, for example, overcoming the embarrassment or awkwardness caused by a colostomy or catheter. Fear of rejection because of physical difference will often inhibit people from embarking on relationships.

People with learning difficulties may need advice or guidance on what is appropriate (or inappropriate) behaviour in public. They are often a vulnerable group, particularly in community settings. This is often a cause of great concern to their parents or carers.

Partners may often also be carers of people with disabilities and switching roles between 'nurse' and 'lover' can cause problems for both people in such a relationship. When a person becomes disabled, both they and their partner may need help to grieve for the loss of their previous sexual relationship. Professionals may often need to give permission and encouragement to couples to explore the possibilities and make choices in terms of their future physical and sexual relationships. Emotional and psychological needs are often linked to practical problems.

Practical guidance on overcoming disabilities

Individuals with disabilities will also need advice on how to overcome some of the practical difficulties associated with specific disabilities and on how to achieve a satisfactory sex life.

Mechanical problems because of restricted or impaired movement due to arthritis, limb deformities or paralysis may be overcome by planning sexual activity and by using pillows to allow comfortable positions to be achieved. Experimentation with different positions may allow vaginal penetration. If the man is unable to acquire an erection then the options such as penile implants, penile injections, erection aids or sex aids should be discussed. Other practical advice may be given on how to achieve intercourse with an in-dwelling urinary catheter, for example whether it can be blocked off. If continuous drainage is essential then strategies for having intercourse without blocking the tubing need to be worked out. Other simple advice may include emptying a colostomy bag before intercourse or timing pain relief medication to ensure maximal effect when intercourse is planned.

Fulfilling sexual relationships do not have to include sexual intercourse for any group and for some with severe disability, penetrative intercourse may be impossible. People may need advice and guidance on developing other techniques for giving and receiving sexual pleasure such as stroking, massage, oral sex and masturbation. Couples will need to explore possibilities and make personal choices that are right for them. Useful leaflets are available from SPOD (see *Further reading*, page 14).

Contraception

Physical and mental disabilities only infrequently affect fertility so advice about contraception and prevention of sexually transmitted infections must be available. Equally, a person with disability may want to plan a pregnancy, so needs to have access to wide ranging pre-conceptual counselling and preparation. Close liaison is important between the clinician and other agencies for parenthood.

A full range of contraceptive services needs to be offered, while taking into account the constraints of any medical condition. Chapter 6 of this handbook (page 83) is based on the

WHO document *Improving access to quality care in family planning* (see *Further reading*, page 14). This provides helpful guidance by reviewing the medical eligibility criteria for selecting contraceptive methods, particularly for those with complex medical problems. Individuals can, all too often, be denied a method of contraception for ill founded reasons. Listed below are some of the chronic medical conditions in which there is no evidence that the combined oral contraceptive (COC) causes deterioration:

- multiple sclerosis
- rheumatoid arthritis
- Hodgkin's disease and non-Hodgkin's lymphoma
- leukaemia
- thyrotoxicosis
- renal dialysis
- asthma
- HIV/AIDS
- myasthenia gravis
- sarcoidosis

Chronic medical conditions which would be affected by COC include:

- systemic lupus
- diabetes with arterial complications – consider progestogen-only pill (POP)
- sex steroid dependant cancers
- long-term immobilisation

Consultations often need different communication methods such as the use of simple diagrams or audio recordings of method information. Such consultations may take more time, possibly requiring several consultations before decisions are reached. Where a patient may not be able to give informed consent, there may be ethical and legal considerations. The book *Sex and the law* (see *Further reading*, page 14) offers useful guidance. Individuals with profound learning difficulties will usually be seen with a parent or carer. At all times it is essential to respect and protect the patient's best interests, even if these may conflict with the wishes of parents or carers. When areas of conflict arise, involvement of other colleagues concerned with the welfare of the individual will often help to resolve difficulties.

Hormonal contraception can often be manipulated to ease some of the practical problems women with learning difficulties experience with menstruation. The combined pill is often an option giving good cycle control with the relief of dysmenorrhoea and may help with pre-menstrual mood fluctuations[26,27]. The achievement of amenorrhoea with depot medroxyprogesterone acetate (DMPA) can be of considerable benefit to the person with restricted mobility or profound learning difficulties[28,29]. Fears of causing affective disorders or mood changes with DMPA have not been substantiated by any studies. Westhoff's study showed that there was little evidence of increasing depression with long term use of DMPA and no short term effect on mood. Therefore, a woman at risk of depression should not be denied this method particularly when the effects of unintended pregnancy on her mental well-being are considered.

Is there a need for special provision?
Women and men with physical, learning and/or mental disabilities may find it difficult to access mainstream services because:

- they do not know where and when services are provided
- they find the physical location of services difficult to access
- they lack the empowerment to access services

It should be possible for people with disabilities to seek sexual health provision from main stream services as long as the provider ensures that information in practice leaflets describes how to access services, making it clear whether disabled access is possible, and if not how to make alternative arrangements with the practice or clinic. In cases where mobility difficulties cannot be overcome then a domiciliary service, such as those provided by some community services, could be offered by GPs with the help of their practice nurse.

part 7

the sexual health needs of gay men, lesbians and bisexuals

Identifying the need

The spread of HIV in the UK has done much to highlight the importance of meeting the sexual health needs of those most at risk of HIV infection. Men who have sex with men form the largest proportion of new AIDS cases each year. In 1993, 63 per cent of cases were in this category. However, new reports of HIV infection among this group have not increased since 1991.

How accessible are existing services?

Studies of GUM clinic use, general practitioner services and dental services highlight perceived deficiencies in existing primary care[30]. These include:

- difficulty of access
- negative/judgmental staff attitudes
- lack of confidentiality
- overall insensitivity

However, in one study 84 per cent of gay men regarded their GP as an appropriate source of safer sex advice. In the same study 44 per cent of men who knew themselves to be HIV positive had not informed their GP of their status despite one third of them having seen their GP in the previous 12 months. This may demonstrate a lack of confidence in sharing such information with their GPs. The evidence suggests that if gay men, lesbians and bisexuals are confident of a non-judgmental sympathetic and confidential consultation then primary care would be an appropriate source of sexual health care and education.

Outreach work

Most health authorities in the UK support outreach workers who visit gay/lesbian venues to provide individuals with information about sexual health and how to access locally available services. Outreach workers will also try to reach those who do not use services such as young gay men, men new on the 'scene' and men who use the public sex environment in order to meet sexual partners. Relatives and friends may also need counselling and support in order to come to terms with an individual's sexuality. Another responsibility of outreach workers should be to build healthy alliances with statutory and non-statutory agencies to raise awareness of services available. It is helpful to have leaflets with lists of agencies that can provide help and support to this group of people. For further details, see *Further reading* (page 14) and *Useful organisations* (page 191).

IMPROVING ACCESSIBILITY OF SERVICES

- **never make assumptions when taking a history, talk to patients about their partner rather than wife/husband/girlfriend/ boyfriend**
- **Allow patients the opportunity to disclose sensitive information**
- **Ensure that practice or clinic literature stresses confidentiality and non-judgmental attitudes when describing how the practice or clinic deals with personal issues**
- **Ensure good links with main stream GUM services which will be aware of any outreach work aimed at these groups of individuals**
- **Ensure all clinic staff have sufficient knowledge and skills to provide a sensitive, non-judgmental and appropriate service**

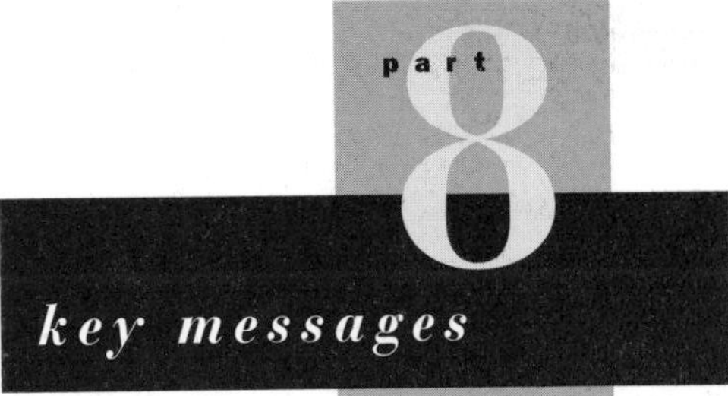

Young people

- **Assess local needs**
- **Timing and location of clinics should attract young people**
- **Informal/no appointment sessions**
- **Confidentiality/anonymity essential**
- **Links to local outreach work**
- **Initial and ongoing advertising of session**
- **Liaise with other agencies to develop a strategic approach**

People with disabilities

- **Ask the question 'How would a disabled patient know that a service exists?'**
- **How easy is it for a disabled person to access your service?**
- **When dealing with disabled people adopt an holistic approach**
- **If you do not have the skills to deal with a person's problem, involve a colleague who does possess those skills**
- **Ensure staff have had appropriate training**
- **Ensure sufficient flexibility to allow for home visits when appropriate**

Gay men, lesbians and bisexuals

- **Never make assumptions in consultations**
- **Allow patients opportunities to disclose sensitive information**
- **Ensure staff are trained to be understanding and non-judgmental in their attitudes**
- **Ensure confidentiality**
- **Develop and maintain liaison with other sexual health service providers**

- ***Handicapped married couples***
  Craft A and Craft M
  Routledge & Kegan Paul, 1979
- ***Learning to love (booklets),***
  Frasier J
  Brook Advisory Centres, 1991
- ***Mental handicap and sexuality***
  Craft A
  EJ Costello, 1987
- ***Sex and the law: A brief guide for staff working with people with learning difficulties***
  Gunn MJ
  Family Planning Association, 1996
- ***Sexual options for paraplegics and quadriplegics***
  Mooney TO, Cole, and Chilgren RA
  Little, Brown and Co, USA, 1975
- ***Sexuality and young people with learning difficulties. A booklet for parents and carers***
  Aran K
  Special Needs Sexuality Project, 1995

SPOD (Association to Aid the Sexual and Personal Relationships of People with Disability) leaflets

- No 2 ***Physical handicap and sexual intercourse: positions for sex***
- No 3 ***Physical handicap and sexual intercourse: methods and techniques***
  (see *Useful addresses*, page 192)
- **Video**
  Living, loving and ageing
  (about elderly people's sexual health)
  Age Concern
  (see *Useful organisations*, page 194)

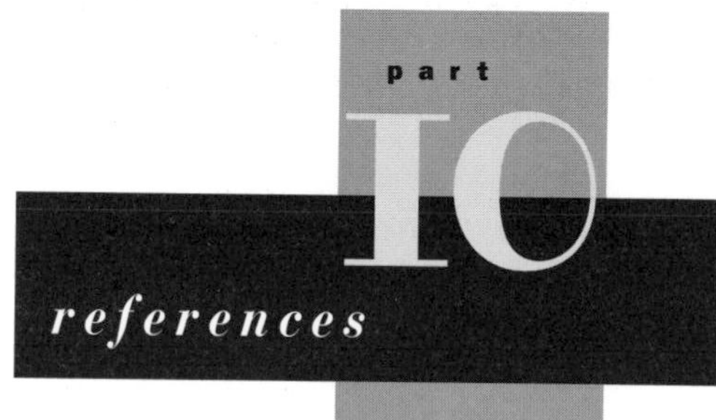

1 ***A sexual health service under one roof: setting up sexual health services for women***, Greenhouse P, ***Journal of Maternal and Child Health, 19,*** 1994, 228-33

1a ***Contraception in western Europe: a current appraisal***, Ketting E (ed), 'Family Planning in Western Europe: an overview of major issues', Ketting E, Parthenon Publishing, 1990, 1-7

2 ***Executive letter*** EL (90) MB 115, Department of Health, 6 June 1990

3 ***Guidelines for reviewing family planning services: guidance for regions***, National Health Service Management Executive, 1992

4 ***HSC (IS)32***, Department of Health, 1974

5 ***Health of the nation: a strategy for health in England***, Department of Health, HMSO, 1992

6 ***Public health standard data sets***, Office of Population Censuses and Surveys, 1993

7 ***Effective Health Care, 3,*** 1, 1997, 1, NHS Centres Reviews and Dissemination, University of York

8 ***Young mothers***, Phoenix, A Oxford Polity Press, 1991

9 'Comparison of childhood background of teenage mothers and their non-mother peers: a new formulation', Oz S and Fine M, ***Journal of Adolescence, 11***, 1988, 251-61

10 ***Report of the RCOG working party on unplanned pregnancy***, Royal College of Obstetricians and Gynaecologists, 1991

11 ***Gillick v the West Norfolk and Wisbech AHA and the DHSS (1996) Appeal Cases (England) 112***

12 ***The economics of family planning services: a report prepared for the Contraceptive Alliance***, McGuire A and Hughes D, Family Planning Association, 1995

13 ***Teenage pregnancy: prevention and programmes***, Peckham S, Ingham R and Diamond I, Institute for Health Policy Studies, University of Southampton, 1996

14 'The economic value of contraception: a comparison of fifteen methods' Trussell J, Leveeque J and Coenig J, et al, ***American Journal of Public Health, 85***, 1995, 494-503

15 'The cost effectiveness of family planning service provision', Hughes D and McGuire A, ***Journal of Public Health Medicine, 18***, 1996, 189-96

16 'Contraceptive services for teenagers: do we need family planning clinics?' Allaby M, ***British Medical Journal, 310***, 1995, 1641-43

17 ***Family planning and pregnancy counselling projects for young people***, Allen I, Policy Studies Institute, 1991

18 ***Confidentiality and people under 16: joint guidance***, BMA, Brook, FPA, GMSC, HEA, and RCGP, 1993

19 'The needs of people with disability', Cooper E, ***British Journal of Family Planning, 21***, 1995, 31-32

20 'Knowledge, attitudes and behaviour related to Sexuality in Adolescents with chronic disability', Cromer BA, Enrile B and McCoy K, et al ***Developmental Medicine and Child Neurology, 32*** 1990, 602-10

21 'Sexual behaviour of adolescents with chronic disease and disability' Suris JC, Resnick MD and Cassuto N, et al, ***Journal of Adolescent Health, 19***, 2, 1996, 124-31

22 'Prevalence of self-reported erectile dysfunction in people with long term IDDM' Klein R, Klein BEK and Lee KE, et al, ***Diabetes Care, 19***, 1996, 135-41

23/24 'Multiple sclerosis and sexual dysfunction – a review', Dupont S, ***Clinical Rehabilitation, 9***, 1995, 135-41

25 'Sexual medicine' Maurice WL, ***Journal of the Canadian Medical Association, 132***, 1986, 1123-25

26 'Depo-Provera for PMT' Robinson W, et al, ***British Journal of Family Planning, 18(1)***, 1992, 29

27 'Depo-Provera for PMT' Cooper E, ***British Journal of Family Planning, 18(3)***, 1992, 97

28 'Depot-medroxyprogesterone acetate contraception: metabolic parameters and mood changes' Westhoff C, ***Journal of Reproductive Medicine, 41(5)***, 1996, 401-6

29 'Depression in users of Depo-medroxyprogesterone acetate, Westhoff C, et al, ***Contraception, 51***, 1995, 351-54

30 ***Men who have sex with men***, Health Education Authority, 1995

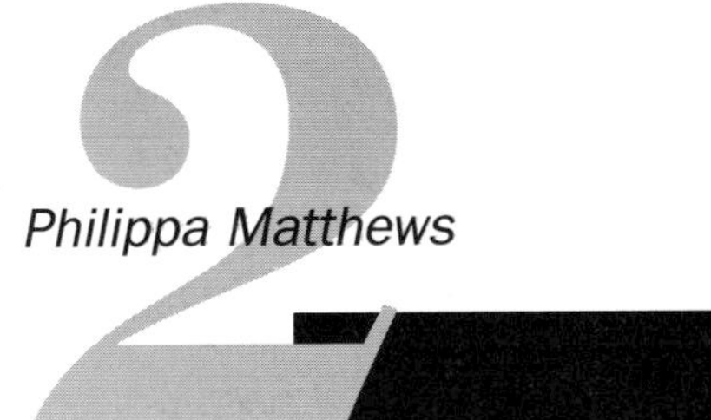

Philippa Matthews

chapter two

sexual history taking in primary care

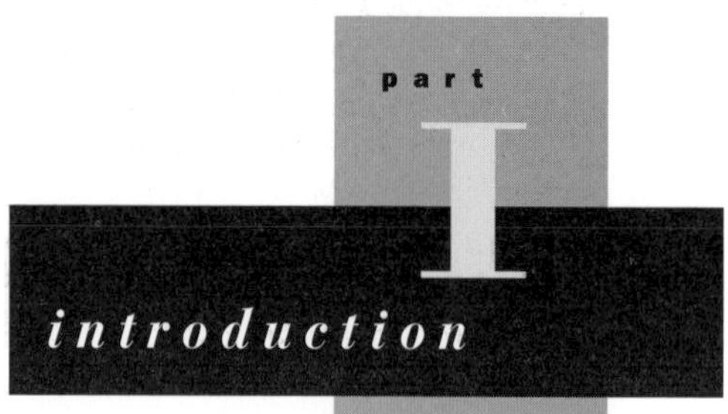

Taking a competent history is the key to the clinical process, especially in primary care. Medical students are taught to take comprehensive histories from patients as they progress through their clinical attachments. Nurses learn to take histories less formally, by identifying which questions they need to ask in order to practice safely (for example, asking about contra-indications to the combined contraceptive pill).

Generally, the question list that makes up a history is taught to medical students in the context of the body system to which they relate. They learn which presenting stories and which answers are significant. When working in general practice, a doctor will sort and select questions that are appropriate to a given consultation, often changing track as the history unfolds. This skill depends on having a view of comprehensive histories, even if they are relatively rarely needed in their entirety. The hypotheses then formed on the basis of the history dictate which system or systems will be examined – or indeed if the patient will be examined.

In sexual health work, processes have evolved differently, and to the particular disadvantage of those who work in primary care (and therefore their patients). When we learnt to examine male genitalia we were taught to ask questions about urinary flow and rising in the night to pass water. When we learnt to examine female genitalia, we were taught to ask about the menstrual cycle, and possibly also about pain and discharge. However many of us were not taught how to assess the risk of a patient having a sexually transmitted infection; what many of the symptoms of infections are; or how to ascertain if there were psychosexual problems. Indeed we could generally avoid the subject of sex altogether – somehow sanctioned by our training.

We can argue that primary care is the most accessible part of the health service to many groups in need of high quality sexual health promotion and care[1,2]. It makes little clinical sense to divide up the clinical issues that relate to sexual health. Both risk of infection and psychosexual problems may affect contraceptive choice, risks or effectiveness. Psychosexual problems may place a patient at risk of infections or unintended pregnancy. Established sexually transmitted infections may give symptoms we misinterpret. Indeed we may even exacerbate the effects of infections through our own clinical interventions. In primary care, our patients may present with problems totally unrelated to sexual health whilst they carry a 'hidden agenda' of a sexual health issue. Thus our traditional gynaecological and contraception training may have left us with too narrow a view of sexual health. Through it men are virtually left out of the picture.

part

2

the role of primary care professionals

Does the GP have a role in the diagnosis or management of sexually transmitted infections (STIs)? In one study of about 19,000 adults, the majority of people with high risk lifestyles for STIs had not attended a genitourinary medicine (GUM) clinic[1]. We may hope that people with symptoms of STIs will present to GUM clinics. However the situation has become far more complex since the extent of infections with either atypical – or no – symptoms has become more clear. Chlamydia and gonorrhoea can both cause pelvic inflammatory disease (PID) with low grade symptoms and little discharge. Chlamydia can cause peri-hepatitis and peri-appendicitis or menstrual abnormalities.

As our ability to test for infections in primary care improves with improved technology, it becomes less and less clear how we can avoid clinical involvement at some level. If patients with atypical symptoms are more likely to present in primary care (rather than self-refer to GUM) then we as GPs need be particularly well-informed as to the variety of subtle or insidious presentations. We must judge whether dysuria is due to a urinary tract infection (UTI) or an STI; whether menorrhagia requires gynaecology referral, thyroid function tests or chlamydia swabs; whether seborrhoeic dermatitis requires a consideration of HIV – or topical treatment alone. We cannot simply delegate this work to a GU clinic, even if we could assume that all patients referred on would attend. However GPs may find they do not have the skills to use the history to its full diagnostic advantage in these contexts.

Asymptomatic infections also affect the picture. The list of sexually transmitted infections that may have no symptoms is now recognised to be long. Genital herpes, syphilis, trichomoniasis, hepatitis B, genital warts, papilloma virus, HIV and chlamydia are all infections that can be sexually transmitted from a person who is entirely symptom-free. And yet many of these infections can have very serious physical consequences. This recognition should give us a particular impetus to maximise sexual health promotion work in primary care. If patients carrying asymptomatic STIs will be using primary care, how can we identify when our clinical input may help?

Practice nurses may play an important part through sexual health promotion. This is now often seen as part of their role through their work in many areas, ranging from contraception to travel advice. Through this work, some practices are beginning to address issues of sexual health and contraception for men. Many practices are taking on chlamydia testing – case finding or screening in some groups – in primary care. They are involved in condom distribution and Hepatitis B immunisation. They understand smears may detect infections – or that smears may be avoided for psychosexual reasons. For all of this work to be handled well, sexual history taking skills must be effective. However practice nurses may also find themselves poorly equipped to do this. In addition the training they undergo that relates most closely to sexual health work may have involved clinical attachments which had no – or few – male patients.

There is already great debate about the costs of these divisions within sexual health[3]. There are even encouraging signs of change amongst some of the specialties concerned. Some GU clinics are providing contraception. Family planning clinics are growing more aware of the importance of sexually transmitted infections. GU clinics are co-operating with gynaecologists to develop protocols for the management of PID. The National Association of Family Planning Nurses has changed its name to the National Association of Nurses for Contraception and Sexual Health.

Thus in primary care we need to consider our training needs carefully. Those of us involved in teaching doctors and nurses bound for primary care need to work to avoid any unhelpful perpetuation of the specialist divisions that we inherited. We must forge an inclusive view of sexual health promotion and care that is appropriate to our needs in primary care. We must also re-examine the points of interface between ourselves and others involved in sexual health work, in order to influence the quality of both training and service provision.

The context and content of the sexual history

The scope and quality of the sexual history taken from a patient will greatly influence clinical practice in the consultation. Effective history taking is about competent clinical care. A sexual history outline may appear in black and white, but would lose its assets entirely if taken as a questionnaire to be run through with the patient. Communication skills are paramount here. The current focus on communication skills training in general practice will help sexual history taking skills. Practice nurses may find communication skills training harder to access. If one point is to be made, it should be that about the value of open questions, ie those which do not imply a 'yes/no' answer. Communication skills are also discussed in Chapter 10 (see pages 148 and 149).

Our own attitudes can also be highly influential on the course and outcome of a consultation.

Cultural issues may be of great importance. If assumptions are avoided, and patients allowed to self-define, then there should be few problems encountered, even when working with someone from a culture with which one has no familiarity or experience. An awareness of the important issues of a culture should be balanced against the needs of a patient – particularly a young person – who may hold a differing individual view. These issues are addressed in greater detail in Chapter 1.

Language barriers may be much more pertinent – not least because family members are so often used to interpret. Appropriate interpretation services are essential in sexual health work, however hard this may be to achieve in practice.

There are some important contextual issues which affect sexual history taking in primary care. One is the problem of raising sexual health issues 'out of the blue'. The other is when trying to deal appropriately with an accompanied patient. These situations need to be managed before a sexual history can be taken.

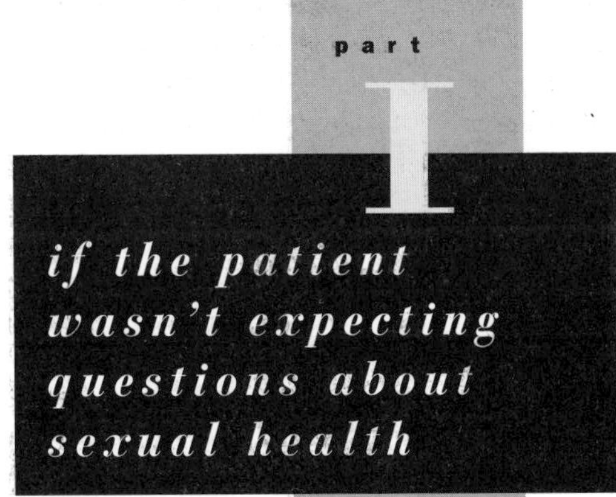

part I

if the patient wasn't expecting questions about sexual health

In most consultations which relate to sexual health it is apparent to the patient that questions about their sexual life are appropriate and necessary. Sometimes this realisation comes as we move through the 'safer' areas, for example establishing their domestic status. However there are occasions in primary care when we wish to negotiate a transition to this area of questioning, and we have the impression that this may come 'out of the blue' to the patient.

A practice nurse may wish to move on to sexual health promotion as part of a new patient check, or a GP may suddenly realise that HIV disease is on the list of differential diagnoses.

The new patient check for a young person:

'Now I'd like to move on to sexual health. At our practice we want to try and help young people avoid sexual health problems or concerns – so would you mind if I asked you a few questions?'

'We have condoms available at this practice. Would it be OK if I asked you a few questions to see if you need them, or what type you might need?'

The (unaware?) patient who may have HIV:

'Have you had any thoughts or worries about what might be causing your symptoms?'

This old favourite question of general practice may help you out here – some patients of course are brimming with concern that this could be HIV related, and this is their chance to open up. This approach works gratifyingly often.

'I am wondering if your symptoms could be due to any kind of sexually transmitted infection – do you think you could be at risk?'

This question is intended to open up the area – the patient's own assessment of their risk may be based on lack of understanding of what is risky, or may simply reflect denial. It should not be accepted by the doctor at face value. However the question can be a useful first step for you.

case study

A GP was called out to see a patient, James, who was a temporary resident staying with his mother. James was a 22 year old media studies student. He was very febrile with a bad sore throat. On examination the GP established that apart from his inflammed throat, James had a blotchy trunkal rash, and oral and perianal ulceration. The GP became concerned that James had HIV seroconversion illness. James's mother was not in the room.

'Did you have any thoughts about what the cause of this is?'

'Just a sore throat isn't it?'

The GP left a pause, weighing up whether he could somehow arrange to see James again. But James spoke again

'You're not thinking of HIV are you?'

'Why do you bring up HIV?' asked the GP

It turned out James had had an HIV positive partner for 5 months. Whilst they had apparently usually used condoms, James seemed a little vague about whether they had all the time. After discussion James said he would like to go to the GUM clinic in his home town to discuss it. The GP pointed out the advantages of early diagnosis if it was HIV. James said it was OK to put the possible diagnosis on the temporary resident card. The GP was surprised at how calm James had been.

part

2

if the nurse or doctor wasn't expecting questions about sexual health

In the primary care context we may get to know patients extremely well over time through problems that have not related to sexual health. It can be difficult or embarrassing for the patient – and perhaps the nurse or doctor – if the patient wishes to raise an issue of sexual health. We may need to make clear that we are prepared to 'change track' onto issues which relate to sexual health at the first cues from the patient that they have questions or a problem.

If embarrassment is unavoidable, it may be best acknowledged:

'I'm glad you felt able to bring this up. Tell me a bit more about it.'

'Don't worry about being a bit embarrassed – we're here to help you with this, just as much as with your diabetes.'

'Obviously after all these years of discussing Tim and his problems, we're both finding it a bit difficult to talk about something as personal as this. But I'm glad you brought it up, and I'm sure we can find a way of helping....'

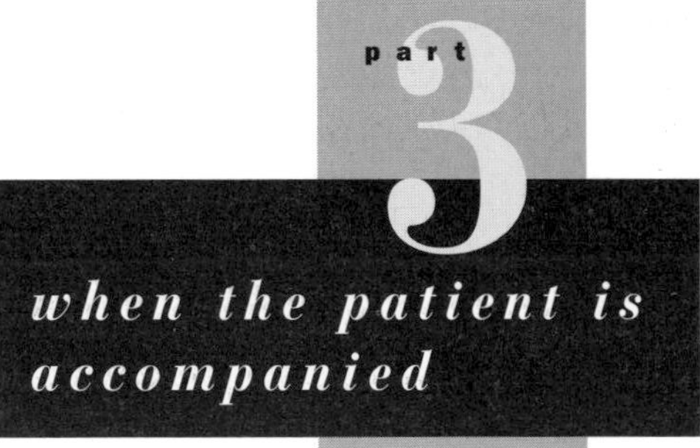

part 3

when the patient is accompanied

Two adults

It is not unusual for patients to be accompanied in primary care. If an adult brings another adult, it may be for a number of reasons:

- it may be for moral support, indicating the patient may view the consultation with some trepidation
- it may be because the two feel that they both have a stake in the problem, or its management
- it may be to introduce the partner to the doctor – it is worth noting that disclosure of sexuality can occur in this way
- the person accompanying may be unwelcome, but has insisted on attending

In most consultations we are likely to clarify the relationship of the pair. However if the consultation moves on to aspects of sexual health, the nurse or doctor may need to check whether the patient would prefer to be alone. The patient may have been unaware that very personal questions would be needed in the assessment of their problem. Or, if the patient had wished to see the doctor alone, but had not been able to negotiate this – it gives them the opportunity to make their preference clear. However, many patients will of course wish their companion to remain. The patient will usually give cues which help us to identify the right course of action.

Male doctors or nurses seeing female patients should consider whether issues of chaperoning arise, if the companion is invited to leave in such a context.

QUESTIONS TO CLARIFY THE RELATIONSHIP

'Come on in. I don't think we've met?....." '.......and your relationship is...?'

'I don't wish to make any assumptions: could I check if you are friends or partners?'

'I'm glad you've brought your friend for moral support – she's welcome. However when I do smear tests I usually like to ask a few quite personal questions so I can check for health problems. Would it be best to have a few minutes alone?'

'To find out the reasons for this sort of problem, some of the questions I should ask you are quite personal. Would it be best if David waited outside?'

'That's fine – if you'd like her to stay in, she stays!'

'So you are clear on our plan then? I'd find it helpful if you could attend the next appointment alone, if that would be OK?'

A young patient accompanied by an adult
When dealing with young people, clinical staff need to be aware of 'Gillick' issues (see page 8), and current guidelines. This awareness affects the way we may handle taking a history and negotiating confidentiality. Service provision issues affecting young people are discussed on pages 5–8. See also the joint guidance issued by the BMA and others[4].

It is clearly ideal if a young person has willingly brought along an involved and supportive adult. It may, however, be very difficult to be sure whether this is or isn't the case. The young person may not imagine that they could be seen alone, or that confidentiality can be protected in the great majority of circumstances if they wish. They may not feel able to indicate that they would prefer the adult to leave. Some doctors and nurses respond to this by routinely asking the accompanying adult to wait outside for a moment, while they establish the wishes of the young person.

(to the accompanying adult)
'At this point I'd like to use my usual routine with young people, whom I like to see alone for a couple of minutes. Could I just ask you to take a seat outside for a moment? And afterwards we'll make sure there is a chance to talk things over.'

(to the young person)
'I realise you may well prefer to have your Mum in with you, but I'd like to give you a chance in case there's anything you'd like to ask?'

'You know that we don't have to tell anyone else about your problems if you don't want us to. The only time is if we think you are in danger of some kind, and we need to talk to others to get the right help.'

'Now let's agree what I can and can't discuss with her when she comes back in.'

It should be made clear to the parent if the young person hadn't any secret agenda items, to support the open relationship.

'Come on in, Mrs Brown. Tracey and I have had a talk, and she's keen you should know there are no secrets. Let's talk things through...'

If there have been secrets, a young person may respond to a strategy of involving the adult then or later. They may feel – perhaps unexpectedly – supported by the doctor or nurse. However, in circumstances where there remain secrets, there is usually some level of discussion at which a parent can be made to feel included again.

part 4

when the patient is unaccompanied

We may wish to see a patient with their partner in order to address sexual health issues. The partner, however, may not come for a number of reasons:

- they may not be registered at the practice, and may not wish to see a doctor or nurse they do not know
- the partner may not wish to attend, perhaps because they view the problem as trivial, or embarrassing, or their fault. They may wish to deny there is a problem, or feel it has nothing to do with them. Or they may think no-one can help
- the patient may not have conveyed effectively the value of a joint attendance, perhaps because of embarrassment, denial, guilt or anger

We should make a clear case for seeing the couple together, and point out what limitations there may be if the patient is seen alone. However it is not uncommon to have to tackle a problem with the patient alone, even when this is far from ideal.

An unaccompanied young person should be made welcome – they may have found it extremely difficult to come and seek help. As discussed earlier in this section, clinical staff should be familiar with young people's rights to confidential care and should understand the legal position with regard to 'Gillick competence' (see Chapter 1, page 8).

Non-clinical staff also need to be aware of young people's rights.

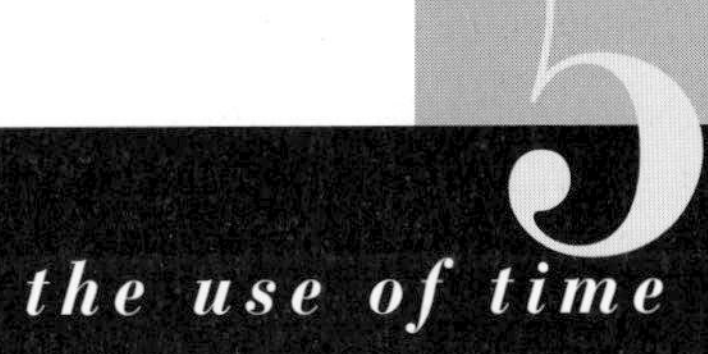

part 5

the use of time

The obvious response of GPs and practice nurses who are being encouraged to take sexual histories is '...but there isn't enough time'. This is clearly always going to be a problem with some patients some of the time. Even when a sexual history has to be taken at some point, we may choose to meet the patient at another time in order to do it, rather than take it at the end of a lengthy 'emergency' surgery or busy clinic. However sometimes the clinical imperatives will demand a sexual history be taken then and there. We will always have to try and prioritise and sort our work in this way.

However, effective sexual history taking saves time, just as effective consultation skills do in other ways. Indeed without it, patients may be seen on many occasions – and even have multiple investigations – before the sexual health agenda is recognised. Nurses who are experienced in sexual history taking report better use of time in procedures such as smear taking. Sexual histories taken as a routine in new patient checks become brief and focused, but responsive to signals from the patient to slow down and explore the issues more carefully.

For both doctors and nurses this is a rewarding area of enquiry, and may do much to enhance satisfaction with the work.

The sexual history has five possible areas of enquiry:

- the social context and relationships
- contraception
- pregnancy, and problems with
- genital tract pathology: STIs, cancers and other
- sexual health promotion

Clearly the areas of enquiry which require most attention will depend upon the patient and the course of the consultation. As with other body system histories, we will rarely use an entire list. We include some suggested questions for those with less experience, and for those who feel a need to change their approach. Our own phraseology will evolve in response to the patients we have, and also the answers and reactions we obtain.

This account of the structure of the sexual history emphasises the areas that are currently taught least well – areas only briefly covered will either be addressed elsewhere in the handbook, or can be found readily in standard texts.

part 6 the social context and relationships

This area of understanding of our patients veers from everyday information about their domestic status, through to areas that may be of a most intimate and private nature, such as psychosexual issues. With some patients there is a natural flow through to these 'deeper' areas, as the consultation progresses. At the other extreme, some patients may consult in primary care for years before making a disclosure or signalling that exploration of more intimate psychosexual areas is appropriate.

The domestic status and current relationship(s)

This area of questioning establishes who lives in the same household as the patient, and the nature of their relationships. This will often lead naturally to a partner history, if appropriate. It may be a time to enquire about children. Questions are most effective if they avoid assumptions of sexual activity, marital status, gender of the partner and monogamy, for example:

'Are you living on your own?'
'Do you have a partner at present?'

SEXUAL ACTIVITY

'Are you in a sexual relationship?'

Young people in particular may feel pressured if health professionals assume that 'everyone is doing it'. We can be just as approachable and in touch with young people, by making this enquiry in a kind and neutral way.

MARITAL STATUS

'How long have you been together?'

Asking someone about a wife or husband may inadvertently imply disapproval to someone who is not married. It is also very likely to silence patients who are not heterosexual. The information needed for clinical reasons relates more to the duration of the partnership and the possibility of other partners, than to marital status. Terms used by the patient, of course, can be readily adopted or responded to.

GENDER OF PARTNER

'Could I just check: is your partner a man or a woman?'

Asking the name of a partner will not reassure the patient that you have considered that it may be a same-sex relationship. Thus it leaves the patient with their dilemma if they are uncertain of your attitudes.

It is best not to start with closed option questions such as 'are you gay?'. Those times when a considerable amount of history has been taken from the patient, and yet the gender of their partner is still not clear, are often the most important to respond to. Issues of confidentiality arise, which will be discussed later.

MONOGAMY

'Do you have any other partners?'
'Does she have any other partners?'
'are you a one-man woman?' '...is he a one-woman man?'

Avoid emotive terms – 'do you think he sleeps around/plays away from home?' etc. Making inappropriate assumptions may render aspects of our patients' lives invisible to us, and this may well compromise our care. Some people use the term 'open relationship' to refer to an agreement that both parties can have other sexual partners. Clearly patients may be unaware that their partner has other partners. Nevertheless it is often helpful if a patient openly expresses doubt about their partner's monogamy, as the issue of infection is then more easily discussed.

case study

Julia is a 42 year old patient with breast cancer, whom I had been caring for since her diagnosis a year before. Mary is 37, and I had been treating her for depression for three months before they finally attended together, and I realised they had been partners for 9 years. They had taken a while to pluck up the courage and I'm sure with hindsight I could have made it easier. The quality of care for both of them has improved enormously now I know – and we can laugh about the times they used to have to come separately.

case study

Tracey used to use a family planning clinic, but came to the practice nurse for a check for her IUD. She was worried that her husband Mark was 'sleeping around'. At the family planning clinic she had wanted to ask for advice about infections, but decided the nurse 'wasn't expecting any problems' and seemed keen just to get on with the check. Tracey had seen the practice nurse before for a smear, and felt she might be able to bring up her concerns. Things worked out, and she and the nurse agreed on some swabs – and also chatted about how Tracey could discuss things with Mark. She went home with some condoms, and an appointment for the following week with the GP.

case study

I remember a patient when I was a GP trainee. Jill was 36 and had attended for some time with lower abdominal pain, and she had implied dyspareunia. I realised with hindsight that although I was sympathetic, the way I asked questions always assumed a sexual relationship between her and her husband. It was therefore not to me, but to one of the partners in the practice that she finally disclosed never having had a sexual relationship – something she considered deeply embarassing and abnormal. My approach to questioning must only have confirmed to her that her problem was indeed unthinkable. I take more care now.

The quality of a relationship

Relationship problems cover a wide span. A 57 year old woman who feels bored and restricted by her long-time partner might present with symptoms suggestive of depression. An 18 year old man who is being beaten up by his older boyfriend might present with anxiety. However such problems may also be linked directly to sexual health in a number of ways. Relationship problems may affect risk taking behaviour for STIs or unintended pregnancy. They may also cast light on the origins of psychosexual problems.

It is worth noting here that some (particularly older) patients understand the term relationship to imply the sexual aspects of their relationship. This may require careful choice of words on your part, and clarification of what the patient means if it is not obvious how they are using the term.

Domestic violence is perhaps the most extreme type of relationship problem, but is common. It frequently goes unrecognised. Pregnant women may be at increased risk of violence[5]. Current advice suggests that doctors should routinely ask all women direct questions about abuse, and that this would be appreciated[6].

Questions about relationships may start in an open way, and then become more targeted.

'How are things going with Shemina?'
'Is there anything you'd like to discuss about that relationship?'
'Have you talked this over with Mike?'
'I wonder, when she said that, how it made you feel?'
'What you said made me wonder whether he had ever treated you badly?'
'Have you ever been hurt or threatened in a relationship?'

case study

Betty is a 53 year old woman who had been trying to pluck up the courage to tell her GP about the intimidation and violence in her marriage for several years. She was quite a regular consulter and she ended up having fruitless investigations for a variety of things. Her GP described a week when she was trying to 'look afresh at old regulars'. 'I'd known Betty for years – in a way I'd inherited her from a partner who left the practice. I realised I'd never taken time to get to know her. I started asking a little more about her life on a day we weren't too rushed. I knew she didn't work, so I started asking about her and Ken: after an awkward start, she opened up. I have such a different view of her now she has told me this story about her violent and abusive marriage. She told me later that sometimes after having a drink she would practice telling me in front of a mirror. Then when she saw me she would be too ashamed and embarrassed, and just didn't feel she had the courage to talk. I think now I just hadn't given her the opportunity. She is still with Ken – she says she couldn't let her sons down. But our own relationship is much more constructive now.'

The partner history

Having made an assesment of the patient's current relationship(s), their partner history may not yet be apparent. This should also be explored, again avoiding assumptions of gender of partner, or of monogamy.

In assessing a patient's risk of having HIV, it may also be appropriate to ask about the sexuality of partners; whether they have used intravenous drugs and about sexual partners or medical treatment abroad.

In taking a detailed partner history – for example to assess risk for STIs – it is worth being aware that issues of rape or sexual abuse may be raised – at least in the patient's own mind. Clinicians should be alert and responsive to cues from the patient, and be careful to avoid insensitive wording. Supportive silence is sometimes most effective when something is hard for the patient to say.

ASKING ABOUT PARTNERS

'Could I just check how long you have been together?'
'Had you had a sexual relationship before that?'
'Was your previous partner also a woman?'
'Are there any other times that you have had sexual intercourse that we need to consider?'

Sometimes a favourite question has to go, when we suddenly realise why it may not be so effective.

case study

Lynn was 21, had a child and was considering having an IUD. Her GP pointed out the risks of the method, and asked her if she was in a steady relationship. 'Oh yes' came her reply, with a reassuring smile. Only later did the GP realise that 'steady' to Lynn meant three months – a record duration for her, about which she felt very cheered. Beware questions about 'steady' or 'stable' relationships!

Sexuality – when do we need to know?

We all have sexuality, and our sense of it may change or evolve through our lives. It is intentionally a broad term to use, and encompasses sexual orientation. In the context of a GU clinic, every patient will be expected to be asked detailed questions about their sexual life. This is not the case in primary care, and we often have to make judgements about whether and when to ask. Are we responding to our agenda, or the patient's?

It is hard to imagine being a good 'family' doctor to someone if we are totally ignorant of the existence of their life partner. In this simple sense, it is important to be aware of the sexuality of our patients. Nevertheless, some patients may have concerns – about our attitudes, or confidentiality perhaps – which may inhibit them from discussing their sexuality with us.

It is worth allowing patients to define their own sexuality in their own terms. For example some men who have had male sexual partners may not identify themselves with the label 'gay' – which they might associate with young men who frequent gay pubs and clubs. Others may see themselves as bisexual. Labels are not generally necessary, although many patients may volunteer them, and it is then a simple matter to respond to and use their own terms. The starting point therefore becomes the questions about the gender of current and past partners. Marital status is not reliable as a quick guide to a patient's sexuality.

The latter is a balance to be struck both with new patients and with regulars. We need to judge – to our best ability – when the sexuality of our patients is not pertinent to the problem being discussed. Patients are likely to withdraw or feel angered if they feel their sexuality is being raised in an inappropriate context.

case study

David was a new patient, a 37 year old manager. He had been attending with stress-related symptoms. He referred to his 'partner' a couple of times, so his GP decided to clarify who this was. His partner was indeed male. David's initial reaction to the enquiry was defensive – almost angry. However, the GP was able to tackle the issues that concerned David: confidentiality, and his fears about her own attitudes. David relaxed a bit, and became open for the first time. It was established that he had a 3 year old daughter from a previous marriage. Because of problems with his ex-wife and her new partner, he had been unable to see his daughter for a year, and was in deep grief. He was in a relationship with Alan, and for both of them, this was their first relationship with a man. After this turning point, David continued to attend with physical symptoms, and began to accept that they usually related to stress, and the loss of a relationship with his daughter. Alan hasn't registered yet, but knows that he is welcome.

case study

Albert is a 48 year old homeless man with alcohol dependency. He developed chronic diarrhoea. After a couple of consultations and some initial investigations, his GP realised that he had not considered HIV disease as a possibility. At some level he had decided Albert was not at risk – perhaps even he had decided Albert was not sexually active. Yet when he began to take a sexual history he found that Albert had had unprotected anal intercourse with several different male partners. It transpired that he was not HIV positive. However his GP became more ready to take sexual histories, rather than rely on hunch.

Psychosexual issues

It is central to our work in primary care, that patients often have hidden agendas. We are trained to be responsive to cues from the patient, and we may feel a need to ascertain if there are psychosexual problems. As a general rule it is better not to ask about specific things, such as pain. Trying to give the patients a feeling that we have time to listen is often hard to do, but likely to be much more rewarding with those who are reticent. Our approach to questions will of course be informed by any cues thus far.

If an agenda is completely hidden, we can at least work in ways that help the patient. This is particularly appropriate when the consultation appears to centre around a task – giving out condoms, doing a smear or prescribing the contraceptive pill. A brief open question can lead to the disclosure of important problem areas in some of our patients.

Even an initial exploration of psychosexual problems may lead to the patient making an important disclosure – such as rape, or sexual abuse in childhood. Alternatively the patient may become upset without disclosing why. Health professionals do not have to have ready solutions, they just need to show that they have heard, and to show care and support. Handling the moment of disclosure is the important thing – finding appropriate support can often be done after the consultation.

'How's sex?'
'Anything you wanted to ask about sex?'
'You look very upset. There may be things that you are uncertain whether to tell me or not. Whether you do or don't, I am here to help you.'

These questions may discourage disclosure, but acknowledge support and concern. Appropriate referral can then later be discussed with the patient.

'It seems there is something you are finding it very difficult to say…' will tend to encourage disclosure.

'It has obviously upset you telling me about what [your father] did. I'm glad you did, because it is the first step to helping you.'

case study

Janet is a practice nurse who attended a training session on sexual history taking. She started asking patients who attended for smears a brief open question: 'How's sex?'. A month later, Janet talked about how her change in practice had gone: 'I found I became more confident in asking after a while – I think I was scared I might get answers that I wouldn't be able to deal with: though now I'm not sure what I was so scared of. Most patients seem to appreciate the asking, but don't have a problem. One patient in my first week went on to describe deep dyspareunia, and so I suggested she saw the GP, and it turned out she had PID. In another patient the question lead to her disclosing childhood sexual abuse – just the telling seemed to help her. I asked her to come back because I wanted to ask advice about where she can get counselling if she wants it. I feel I'm doing a much better job now – to think I used to talk about the weather because I thought it made the patients relax! – that seems like a wasted opportunity, now'

Sexual practices – when do we need to know?

Asking patients about their sexual practices is often seen as a particularly difficult thing. There are a few situations in primary care when it is essential.

ASSESSMENT OF RISK OF HAVING AN STI

When assessing someone' s risk of having an STI – particularly HIV – it may be appropriate to enquire about sexual practices. It should not be imagined that if the sexuality of a patient is known, that their sexual practice can be assumed. Many gay men do not practice anal intercourse, and a significant minority of heterosexual couples do. Assessing sexual practices in lesbian relationships will help in forming a view of the likelehood of transmission of infection – for example through shared sex toys. There is some preliminary evidence that herpes, trichomonas and human papilloma virus (HPV) may be transmitted woman to woman. Bacterial vaginosis may be more common in lesbian than in heterosexual women attending a GU clinic[7].

Appropriate barrier protection should be recommended to those assessed as being at risk of STIs (see *Use of condoms and other barriers,* page 36).

ASSESSMENT OF PSYCHOSEXUAL PROBLEMS

When assessing sexual practices in this context it is again important to avoid assumptions about what is actually happening, and to bear in mind that the patient might be very ill-informed about their, or their partner's, anatomy.

In all these circumstances there is a need to ensure that patients understand the terms you use, and also that you have the correct understanding of terms patients use. This is best actively judged from the outset. If a patient uses a term with which you are not familiar, they are unlikely to mind if you ask them to explain what they mean, as long as they feel reasonably secure. We usually respond to patients' cues that there are misunderstandings growing. Similarly, it is often instinctively clear when we are communicating effectively, and it is not appropriate to persistently clarify definitions.

'Could I ask some questions about your sexual activity? It will help us decide if you are at risk of infections or not.'
'Could I just clarify what sex involves for you and your partner? It may help me understand why you are having some problems?'
'Do you have anal intercourse?'
'I think you may not have understood me when I used the word 'ejaculate' – shall I try and make myself a bit more clear?'
'I'm afraid I'm not sure what that means – could you explain it to me?'

case study

Heather is a practice nurse in a condom distributing practice. In her first week a man came in for a new registration check, and asked for some condoms. 'I nearly died', Heather said later, 'I knew he'd need stronger condoms if he practiced anal intercourse, but I just couldn't pluck up courage to ask him. In the end I showed him the condom tray, and said 'These stronger condoms and lubricant are for people who have anal intercourse – do help yourself to the type you need'. I was extremely embarrassed and busied myself by clearing away some things while he chose! Since then I've become a lot more confident – getting started was really the only difficult bit'

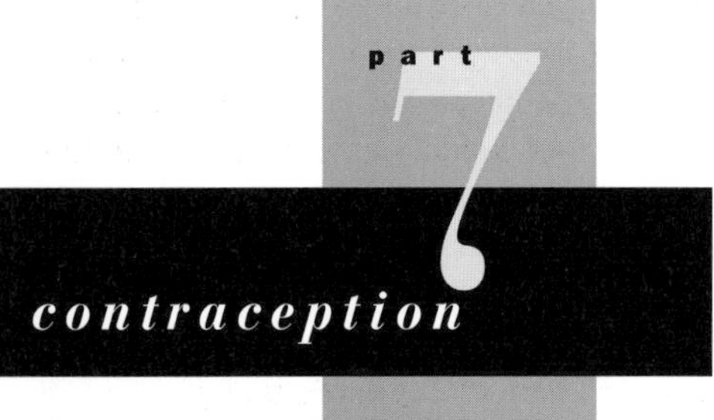

Initial questioning is frequently of a more open nature, as we establish the level of knowledge our patient has, and what opinions they have as to their preferred contraceptive choice. We may review their experiences of different methods, and make judgements about their ability to use them.

We may also ask questions in order to test out our own ideas about an appropriate form of contraception for our patient, and to minimise its risks. Questions will cover contraceptive history, menstrual history and history of any pregnancies. They are also intended to seek out relative and absolute contra-indications to forms of contraception (see Chapter 6).

The significance of STIs should not be overlooked when the choice of contraception is being considered or reviewed: contraceptives may play a role in the prevention or exacerbation of STIs.

Relationship or psychosexual problems may also affect contraceptive choices or a patient's ability to use them. A man may avoid condom use because they once caused him to lose his erection. A woman may avoid using a diaphragm as an option as she believes that she shouldn't touch her genitalia. A man's refusal to use a condom may characterise a violent or abusive relationship.

Men and women who attend for condoms will need at least one opportunity to discuss any aspects of condom use that may concern them. We should not make any assumption that they can use condoms correctly – whilst we must also judge when people know, and don't wish to be 'lectured' . Men who use condoms and have sexual relationships with women may also appreciate information about emergency contraception for their partners.

'Quite a few people who get condoms here like a chance to talk over how to use them safely – would you?'
'Did you know that we provide emergency contraception here if a condom splits or comes off – or if you didn't use one? You have/your partner has up to three to five days depending on the method.'

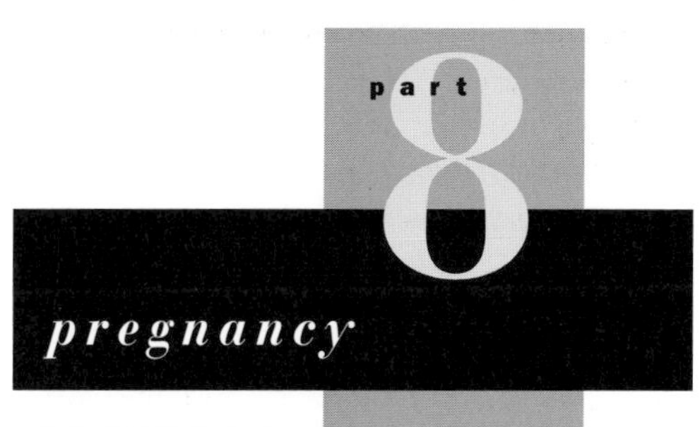

Many questions to sexually active female patients may relate to the exclusion or confirmation of pregnancy, or assessing the likelihood of problems with an early pregnancy. Again, our training is often more thorough in this field, and we are better versed in the best questions to ask.

Questions relate to previous pregnancies, the menstrual cycle, contraception type and use, symptoms of pregnancy and symptoms that may suggest an ectopic or other pregnancy problem.

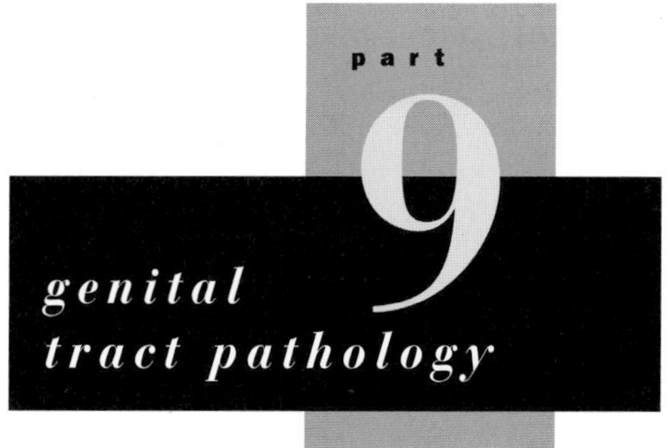

STIs

The key elements to a risk assessment for having an STI are

- partner history
- sexual practices
- a past history of an STI

The first two areas of questioning are considered earlier in this chapter.

We should not collude with a patient's own overall assessment of risk – which may be based on denial or misunderstanding. We will need to ask in more depth.

The genitourinary medicine model of risk of STI ('everyone is at risk') is extremely useful, but perhaps works a little less well for primary care. Some of our patients are indeed not at risk of having an STI, and their menorrhagia or dysuria or discharge must be due to something else, simply because they have never been sexually active. In primary care many patients who say they have never been sexually active will be believed by us, presumably often correctly if we have good mutual rapport and trust. Other patients will perceive themselves as having no risk of having an STI (perhaps making assumptions of monogamy of their partner). Again, we may feel with some of our patients that extensive questioning of these assumptions of their lifetime partner would be insulting. We might seem, for example, to be offending religious beliefs, or inappropriately questioning a lifetime relationship the patient is trying to tell us is close and trusting. A gay man might feel insulted to be considered to be at risk of having HIV or in need of hepatitis B immunisation if he is well informed and at no risk of having these infections.

Our decision in some instances and after careful enquiries, to believe our patients, or occasionally to overlook outside chances of an STI, may affect clinical choices. For example we may feel we should not swab or test for STIs in these situations – perhaps before fitting an IUD, or in investigating a woman who clinically appears to have vaginal candidiasis.

Conversely the process of taking a careful risk assesment will often demonstrate to patients who thought they were not at risk of having an infection that they are – and so the need for investigation may become obvious.

These questions could lead to taking a partner history, and enquiring about sexual practices:

'Did you know you can have an infection without knowing about it?'

'Your symptoms could be due to a number of things, one of which might be a sexually transmitted infection. Is that possible?'
'Could I ask a few more questions so I can be sure that you are right to rule that possibility out?'

The following questions help further in the exploration of the patient' s own views on their past and current risk of acquiring infections:

'Have you ever been treated for a sexually transmitted infection?'
'Have you ever thought you might have a sexually transmitted infection?'

Answers to questions about a past history of STIs may be both diverse and helpful:

'Nothing really, just gonorrhoea and warts last summer'
'Well that was why I chucked him – I got an infection, so I said that's it'
'Oh yes – and now I go every 6 months to the clinic, I call it my MOT'
'Well I did get tests last year, but I never went back for all the results'

All of this is useful information for assessing risk, however we must also be able to recognise and interpret symptoms correctly. This depends upon having good clinical factual knowledge. Particularly in the case of STIs we may find we are ill-informed and poorly served by our training (see Chapter 9 which deals with STIs in more detail). Here the intention is to highlight significant errors or omissions that are common in primary care.

MEN
Male patients, particularly those who are younger, who present with these symptoms should be considered as having an STI until proved otherwise:

- dysuria
- epididymitis
- white cells in the urine (on dipstick or 'sterile pyuria')
- discharge from the penis
- genital or peri-anal sores or warts
- Symptoms suggestive of HIV disease or hepatitis B

Accurate diagnosis should be striven for. Contacts should always be considered.

WOMEN
The more that is learnt about STIs – particularly chlamydia – the more insidious in nature they appear to be. As it is possible for chlamydia to cause complete fallopian tube occlusion in women without having caused any symptoms, we need to have a low threshold for its diagnosis.

We should consider a diagnosis of an STI in women with

- lower abdominal pain
- symptoms suggestive of peri-hepatitis or peri-appendicitis
- dyspareunia
- dysuria, and possibly sterile pyuria
- genital or peri-anal sores or warts
- intermenstrual bleeding, post coital bleeding or menorrhagia
- vaginal discharge
- symptoms suggestive of HIV disease or hepatitis B

Accurate diagnosis should be striven for. Contacts should always be considered.

case study

Sue is a new patient. She is a 26 year old designer. She has had two months of intermittent dysuria, which she has found increasingly troublesome. Her previous GP kept telling her her urine was 'clear', and she felt she wasn't being taken seriously. For this reason she had changed practices. Exploration of her history revealed that she was living with her boyfriend, Tony, in a good relationship of two years' standing. She had had two previous partners. Eight months before registering she had been admitted to hospital with suspected appendicitis, which settled overnight. When the pain niggled on the following week she reported she had been given antibiotics by her GP, but her

partner had not. The pain settled. Last month she had had one episode of intermenstrual spotting.

The clinical picture was considered to be due to chlamydia until proved otherwise – and an endocervical chlamydia culture swab confirmed this. The endocervical swab for gonorrhoea and the herpes simplex virus were both clear. Sue and Tony were both treated, but could not be pursuaded attend the GUM clinic, because they felt the problem was resolved for them. Sue did not know how to contact one of her previous partners, but agreed to take a note with the diagnosis to the other. Tony did not feel his previous partner should be contacted, as they had been mutual first partners.

Sue's symptoms resolved on treatment. She brought up the question of 'damaged tubes'. She now understands she will have to wait and see with regard to her fertility, but remains optimistic.

Cancers and other genital tract pathology

Doctors' clinical training has often served well in identifying such problems. We know the questions needed to elicit the cyclical nature of symptoms due to endometriosis, and we respond appropriately to lumps or pain that may indicate anything from cancer to testicular torsion. Perhaps we are also more at ease because these conditions may have no – or only indirect – connections with sex.

The patient may feel differently – their problem may not relate directly to sex, but it does relate to their sexual organs. They may find it difficult to bring these kinds of symptoms to us. They may feel embarrassed at or scared of the possibility of having an intimate examination – perhaps by a doctor or nurse of the opposite sex. They may feel frightened that their symptoms portend serious illness.

A practice can help to some degree in how it is seen. If new patient checks address prostate or testicular awareness, the practice may be seen as a place where such issues can be raised. Some practices place leaflets on 'sensitive' subjects in accessible areas of the practice, giving them priority when space is short. They reason that it is easier to ask for a leaflet on diet or asthma if one is not on display, than it is to ask for one about testicular lumps.

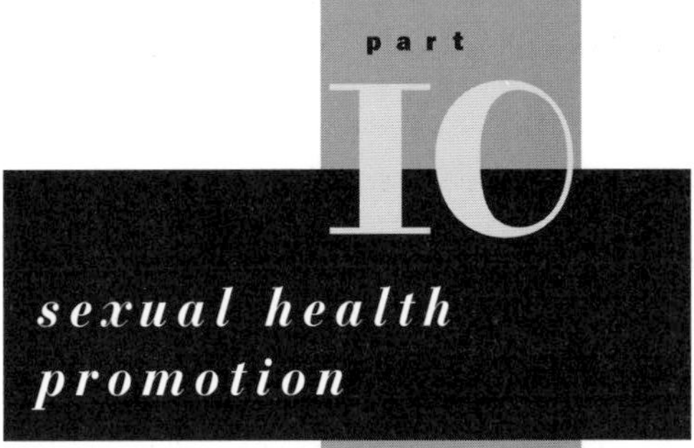

part 10 *sexual health promotion*

After taking a sexual history and addressing a sexual health problem, we will be in an excellent position to give our patient tailor-made information and advice to help them avoid problems.

Alternatively, a patient may attend simply to seek advice about sexual health, without any apparent current problem. A couple might, for example, attend to discuss whether they should have chlamydia swabs – or HIV tests – before stopping their use of condoms. Such patients should be actively supported in their decision-making process. Clinical workers tempted to use the term 'worried well' should be wary they are not covering up their own clinical shortcomings or lack of time!

Finally, sexual health promotion may be initiated by the clinical worker in certain contexts less directly connected with sexual health. For a discussion of these see *Targeting sexual health promotion and care,* page 44.

The prevention of STIs, and limiting their effects

USE OF CONDOMS AND OTHER BARRIERS
This involves the promotion of barriers to infection (such as male and female condoms or dental dams). Contraceptive needs should also be considered. Ensure the patient understands how infections are transmitted, and how to avoid them. Many patients are unaware of the asymptomatic nature of a great number of infections, and also unaware of how some infections such as chlamydia and HIV, can be present for years before causing problems.

Extra-strong male condoms and lubricant will be needed for patients who practice anal intercourse. Condoms should be used on all shared sex toys. Female condoms also offer protection from STIs. Dental dams, which are thin oblong sheets of latex, can be used to prevent the spread of infection during oral sex to cover the anus or female external genitalia. They are available from dental suppliers.

CHLAMYDIA SCREENING OR CASE-FINDING
Many practices now screen for chlamydia in selected patients, using guidelines such as under 25 years, having a change of partner in the last year and attending for a pelvic examination. A skilful sexual history will reveal other patients who may be at high risk of infection. Chlamydia is common, and predictive features are of limited value: a low threshold for testing is appropriate.

Patients undergoing instrumentation of the cervix (such an IUD insertion, termination of pregnancy (TOP), or dilatation and curettage (D&C)) will need especially careful assessment for risk of chlamydia, because of the risk of causing PID. Some practices will screen for chlamydia in this situation. Prophylactic antibiotics may be used, but the implications of not treating the partner in this context are unclear. Use of antibiotics while omitting a test for chlamydia means that patients who are infected remain unaware, thereby missing an excellent health promotion opportunity.

HEPATITIS B IMMUNITY SCREENING
This is important for men who have sex with men, and a blood test is taken to assess hepatitis B immunity and/or carriage. There is evidence that anyone who has multiple sexual partners should also have their immunity checked. Immunisation should be offered to those not immune, and the course should be followed by another check of immunity. This is a good time to ensure that the patient knows how to use condoms if they practice anal intercourse, and that they have the appropriate type, and a lubricant.

HIV TESTING
Recent advances in treatment have led to increasing clinical benefits in identifying who is HIV positive. This is perhaps most clear for women who are pregnant, to offer treatment to decrease the baby's risk of infection.

HIV testing in primary care in this country has been limited, largely because of the conflicting roles imposed upon GPs through involvement in insurance personal medical attendant reports. But increasing numbers of practices are conducting HIV tests. GPs are developing ways to protect patients from discrimination by insurance companies which enquire about past HIV tests (rather than simply aiming to identify those who tested positive). There are hopes that professional and insurance industry guidelines may be changing again to further protect confidentiality and clarify what GPs should do. (See also Chapter 3, *Insurance medical reports... in practice,* page 58.)

Another limiting factor to GP involvement in HIV testing has been the view that only trained HIV counsellors should conduct the tests. However this too is changing: it is now emphasised that lengthy pre-test counselling should not be considered essential. A potentially briefer pre-test discussion should be conducted, with referral on to a specialist counsellor if the circumstances of the individual are 'complex and time consuming'[8], or if a test has proved positive.

Some patients prefer to have the test carried out by their GP, with a familiar face and familiar surroundings. The lack of 'same day' results may not act as a disincentive - particularly now that it is possible to be rather more optimistic about the effectiveness of treatments, and the prospect of a positive result is less extreme.

Involvement in HIV testing nevertheless requires careful thought. GPs taking tests should be be able to conduct a competent pre-test discussion. The possible advantages of GUM clinic testing should be discussed (for example some clinics can give results on the same day).

MANAGEMENT OF CONTACTS OF STIS

The adequate management of contacts of those with STIs is part of sexual health promotion (see Chapter 9, page 142).

The prevention of unintended pregnancies

Promote safe and effective contraceptive use (see Chapter 6). Ensure both men and women are appropriately informed about the role of emergency contraception.

The promotion of healthy pregnancies

This includes awareness of who might benefit from folic acid, the checking of rubella immunity and smoking advice (see Chapter 7, pages 113–114).

The prevention and screening of genital tract cancers and breast cancer

FAMILY HISTORY

Family history may be significant, even if only in the eyes of the patient as a concern that needs to be addressed. Advice from a clinical geneticist may be valuable if the patient has more than one first degree relative affected, particularly if at a young age, and so the details should be explored.

Genital tract cancers that may, in some cases, have a genetic component include:

- ovarian cancer
- endometrial cancer (ask also about bowel, urinary tract or ovarian cancers in relatives because there is an association in some)
- breast cancer (ask also about ovarian cancer in relatives, as there is an association in some). Some postmenopausal breast cancers have a genetic influence
- no genital or urinary tract cancers in men are recognised as having a significant genetic component, including prostate and testicular cancer.

CERVICAL SCREENING

We should check our patients smears are up-to-date, and we may wish to raise factors which affect the risk of cervical cancer such as smoking or human papilloma virus (HPV) infections.

Women who are lesbians should have smears[7]. The reasons for this include the possibility that they may have had sexual intercourse with a man in the past (consensual or non-consensual); they may be at risk of woman to woman spread of HPV; or they may smoke. Lesbian women may not realise that smears are recommended for them, and so reasons should be carefully explained.

HIV testing...in practice

An approach to the HIV pre-test discussion

- **Establish the reasons for testing if the patient has asked.**
  'What made you decide you wanted to come for an HIV test?'

- **Negotiate the reasons for testing if the GP is initiating it**
  See page 36

- **Ensure the patient understands what the HIV antibody test is, what HIV is and what AIDS is.**
  'Tell me what you understand about the HIV test?'
  'What do you understand about the difference between HIV and AIDS?'

- **Risk assessment and inform patient about 'window period' (the 6 to 12 weeks after HIV infection, but before becoming antibody positive)**
  Assess risk of STIs
  Ask about
  - **travel**
  - **IV drug use**
  - **blood transfusions (before 1985 in the UK)**
  - **medical or surgical treatment abroad**
  - **occupational risk**

  Some patients may be reluctant to answer questions as you check through the list, in which case this approach may help:
  'It is not important for me to know exactly what you did, and when you think the last risk occurred. But it is important for you to know. It affects the results, especially if we test too soon after, and the test hasn't yet become positive'

  This will only help if they understand what is or is not risky!

- **Identify patient's main concern, and main benefit from having test**
  'What is your main concern about having a test now?'
  'What is the main advantage for you of having a test now?'

- **Consider the patient's relationships, are there 'key' people?**
  'Have you told anyone you are thinking of having a test?'
  'Is there anyone you would be afraid to tell?'

- **Explore possible reactions to the wait for the result and also to a positive result. Consider both the patient and their 'key' people.**
  'You say you will find it hard waiting for the result. Some anxiety is normal. How can you help yourself?'
  'If the test were positive, how do you think you would react?'
  'If the test were positive, how would David react?'
  'You say you would be desperate. How might you cope with these feelings?'

- **Summarise, and gain consent**
  Some patients may need more time, or to be referred elsewhere
  Clarify how the result will be provided

Points to consider when conducting HIV tests in primary care

- **What steps can be taken to protect confidentiality? What will be recorded in the notes?**
- **Will samples be labelled with the patient's name? Or will another system be devised?**
  Code number systems can be devised with your lab if preferred
  Discuss with the team what approach suits the practice best. Make yourselves aware of current professional guidelines and including those for insurance companies.
- **When will results be given? Will the system work for positive or negative results?**
  Find out how long results usually take – for example some smaller labs may carry out HIV tests on batches once a week.
  Ensure positive results are not going to be given at bad times, such as on a Friday evening.
- **Is any written material about HIV testing needed for the practice?**

Cervical screening...in practice

Guidelines may vary from area to area:

- **cervical cytology is considered unnecessary by some until an under 20 year old has been sexually active for three years**
- **some consider cervical cytology can be discontinued at 55 years**
- **at all ages – including the extremes – other risk factors may affect the decision to screen. These may include a history of genital warts or HPV**
- **women who are lesbians should be offered cervical screening**
- **women who have either HIV or HPV infection will require more frequent smears**

PATIENT SELF-EXAMINATION AND AWARENESS
We may also use the opportunity to address breast awareness, prostate awareness or testicular self-examination.

Developing sexual health promotion and care in practice

There are a number of issues that relate to the provision of sexual health promotion and care in the primary care context. It is advisable to address these as a team, to ensure either some uniformity of approach, or at least an awareness and understanding of individual differences in the team. This may become an opportunity to 'team build' and step back from the workface.

Teamwork issues include:

- **confidentiality**
- **attitudes**
- **consent**
- **targeting sexual health promotion and care**

(See also Chapter 11 on teamworking.)

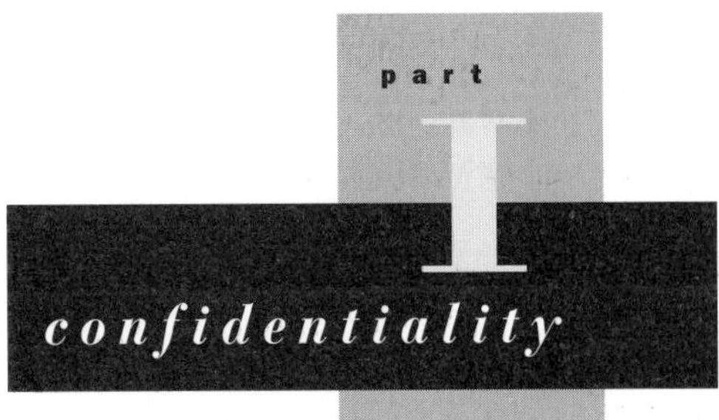

We may take for granted that we provide a confidential service, and yet review by the whole team will almost inevitably reveal areas for improvement.

There are two aspects to confidentiality in primary care: doing, and being seen to be doing.

Ensuring a confidential service

The 'doing' is simply trying to ensure, as far as possible, that your team provides a confidential service. This requires the discussion of confidentiality issues as a team, with the involvement of both clinical and non-clinical staff. The discussion should be informed by an awareness of the legal position, and also of professional guidelines. There is evidence of inconsistency and misinformation in primary care. A Family Planning Association study[9] of 60 practices showed a considerable lack of clarity about the legal position regarding confidentiality and the under 16s.

Many of the main points are covered by a few brief documents, which someone in the team might take time to study if there is uncertainty[4,10,11].

Areas for discussion may include the following:

- Is there information that it is best not to record? What kind of information? Do we all have a similar approach?
- Do the GPs have a similar approach to completing insurance medical reports? Are the practice nurses aware of the implications

for these reports of what they may write in the notes?

- How do we deal with our young patients attending with or without their parents? Are all the team aware of the legal rights of young people seeking care?[4]
- What issues of confidentiality may arise at reception?
- Do we use any forms of note tagging, and, if so, are there implications for confidentiality?
- What issues of confidentiality may arise through the use of the telephone, or the receipt of calls?
- What issues of confidentiality might arise through referral of patients to others? Should a physiotherapy referral mention HIV status?
- Who can access notes or computer records?
- How confidential are the flows of paperwork in the practice?
- How is the issue of confidentiality addressed with either new staff, attached students or other staff in training?

For *Insurance medical reports... in practice* see Chapter 3, page 58.

Making clear a confidential service is provided

This is the 'being seen to be doing'. If your team really does take care to provide a confidential service, what do you do to let your patients know? Is your waiting area or practice leaflet any different from a neighbouring practice who haven't discussed confidentiality issues for years? How could your patients judge the difference? 'Being seen to be doing' simply relates to the problem that there is evidence that many patients have concerns about levels of confidentiality in primary care. Whether founded or not, there are plenty of apocryphal stories about receptionists who are neighbours to aunts and the like. Some groups may have more reason for concern than others. Three-quarters of 15 year olds believe that doctors have to tell parents of a request for contraception[12].

Although we can predict that some groups may have greater concerns about confidentiality than others, we cannot make these predictions at an individual level. Patients may have grave worries that are not fully founded.

case study

Tracey is a practice nurse in a village. A 47 year old woman presented to her with her first episode of vaginal candida, with unusually severe symptoms. The patient thought that thrush was sexually transmitted. In the context of a fairly unhappy marriage, she thought it implied that her husband of 15 years had had another partner. As her husband was a close friend of the GP in the practice, she had avoided coming until the symptoms became unbearable after more than seven weeks. On examination Tracey found clinically typical vaginal candida, though unusually severe. The patients' external genitalia were severely inflammed and excoriated. Speculum examination – which was interupted because of discomfort – gave Tracey a glimpse of typical thick 'clotted' white discharge.

Tracey was able to reassure the patient that candida is not sexually transmitted. She was also able to emphasise that the practice was very conscientious about confidentiality because of the small community it served. This freed the patient to talk more fully about her relationship and fears. They were able to begin to explore her reasons for worrying about sexually transmitted infections, and whether she might indeed have one. The patient revealed a distant relationship with little communication – and nothing concrete to indicate a risk of an STI. After discussion, they agreed that the patient would try to talk with her husband about the relationship, including the possibility of seeing a Relate counsellor. The patient was to return to see the GP after using the prescibed treatment, for further discussion and re-examination.

What can be done to reassure patients that it is safe to talk? A study of HIV positive patients in London found that use of a statement of confidentiality encourages disclosure of HIV status to GPs[13].

An example statement of confidentiality could be:

'We have strict rules about confidentiality, which apply to all our staff. We are especially careful that family members should not be able to learn things about each other, unless consent has been given by the patient concerned. If you have worries about confidentiality, please feel free to discuss it with our doctors or nurses'

You might consider adding:

'If you would like a discussion left off your record, just mention this to the doctor at the start of your appointment'

This is more usually used as an opener by patients, rather than committing us to great omissions from the records. Alternatively:

'If you would like to see our confidentiality policy, please contact our practice manager'.

case study

One practice agreed to have posters made using these statements, and they also included them in the practice leaflet. Patients only occasionally referred to it, but in the few examples it was considered very significant. Those patients used it as an opening to bring up a subject they felt was difficult. There had been concerns about the implications of offering to leave discussions off the record, but most of the patients were less concerned about this once they had had a chance to air their worries. Patients also seem ready to understand that physical problems and tests need to be recorded.

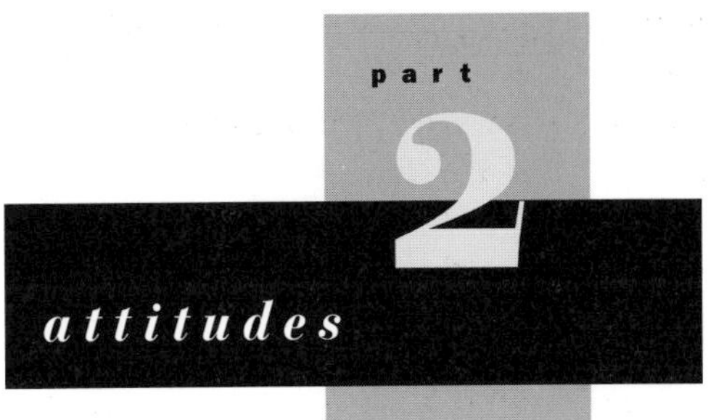

part 2 *attitudes*

Our attitudes as individuals

Many doctors and nurses are used to using a non-judgemental approach with patients, putting to one side their personal views. Involvement in sexual health work seems particularly likely to challenge our abilities to work in this way, and yet if the patient detects disapproval, out ability to work effectively may be lost.

Our professional organisations and the law try to make our responsibilities clear[10,11]. There are few circumstances in which it is considered acceptable to withdraw from clinical involvement the patient (such as referral for terminations of pregnancy) and many when it is not (such as in care of the HIV positive patient or young people). An insidious problem for the patient is if care is not withdrawn but compromised through the attitudes of the doctors or nurses involved. We may – consciously or unconsciously – deter or silence patients who sense they are being judged or disapproved of. And of course, if we unconsciously silence a patient, we have no idea there is a problem.

Reflecting on our own practice may help: for example, when did we last identify a psychosexual problem in a patient? Or when did a patient last disclose that they were in a same sex relationship? Are there consultations which make us feel awkward or embarrassed? We may encounter issues that we need to address as individuals. Our attitudes to aspects of sexual health work may be coloured – or profoundly influenced – by our own experiences. We too may have psychosexual problems. We may never have had a sexual partner. We may be bisexual. We may have suffered sexual abuse or assault.

We may hold an ideal of a single sexual relationship within a life-long marriage. Reflection on our own negative (or positive) reactions may give us insights into their origin.

Most GPs and practice nurses may strive to work in a non-judgemental way. But would their patients know this? Some practices may not have taken sufficient steps to overcome the anxieties that patients may have about the attitudes they may encounter. Young people may doubt the attitudes they feel they are likely to encounter in primary care[12]. Similarly, whilst most gay men may be registered with a GP, many feel their practice has a negative attitude to homosexual men – so many do not inform their GP of their sexuality. Of those who are HIV positive, many choose not to inform their GP[14,13].

case study

Andy attends for travel advice. He is 18, and travelling to an Italian resort for a summer holiday. His mum suggested he saw the nurse because she thought he should ask about 'jabs'. The nurse, Ashti, is keen to target 'sun and sex' health promotion advice for young travellers. Andy is in fact planning to have as many sexual encounters as he can on this holiday. He thinks that if the nurse found this out he would 'get a lecture'. He also thinks Ashti knows his gran well. Will she be able to win him round so she can give him the information (and condoms) that he needs?

Our attitude as a team

Attitudes are worth discussion as a team – although teams might wish to seek a facilitator to ensure this is done constructively. If a primary health care team is interested in trying to provide non-discriminatory care, sexual health may be a useful topic to tackle.

We often form impressions of the attitudes of our colleagues, although they may be incorrect and possibly due to misunderstanding. If a colleague has attitudes that we perceive to be very different to our own, it may be helpful to try to understand their position, particularly so we can try and maximise 'seamless' care.

- How do we feel about the provision of contraception for young people?
- How do we feel about discussing sexual health? Would the gender of the patient make a difference? Or their age? Or if they were in a same sex relationship?
- How do we feel about raising sexual health with a patient 'out of the blue' – for example in a new registration check? Would gender, age or sexuality make a difference here? What phrases do we use to make difficult questions easier?

Many practices include some doctors who will refer patients for terminations, working alongside doctors who will not. In order that this can work well, teams may agree plans to ensure that a smooth handover of patients can occur without the introduction of significant delay. Practice nurses running contraception clinics need to be aware of which doctors will see a patient seeking a termination of pregnancy, and how to access them quickly.

Non-discrimination statements

A study of HIV positive patients in London[13] indicated that a display of a non-discrimination policy might double the number of patients prepared to disclose their diagnosis to staff.

An example non-discrimination statement might be

'We are a service for everyone!
We aim to provide a friendly and helpful service to all.
We hope you will feel able to bring up any health related issue with us, whatever your sexuality, colour or beliefs'

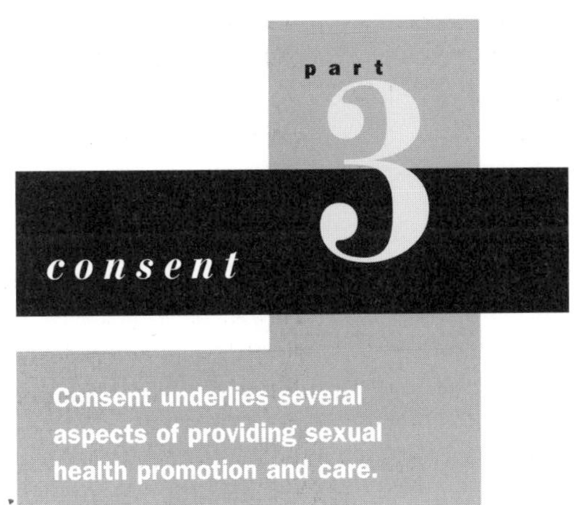

Consent and confidentiality
Consent can underpin confidentiality: where we are uncertain who should know what about a patient, it is best to seek the consent of the patient concerned. If someone who is HIV positive is being referred for a chest X-ray, the patient will usually respond to an open discussion about the merits of informing the radiologist who will be looking at the pictures. The way in which HIV can be referred to on the form can then be negotiated.

Similarly, a young person may be very anxious that we will inform their parents about something without their consent. Once they understand that they are actually in control of the decision, it becomes easier to present and discuss all the options open to them – including, possibly, the involvement of a parent. They have understood that their consent is essential, and the fear is diminished, which frees discussion. Patients respond to an open approach, and will then rarely ignore advice on which choices might compromise quality of care.

Consent for tests for STIs
We are now well aware of the implications of HIV testing, and the need for informed consent. However tests for other STIs can also raise important issues of consent. If we perform endocervical or chlamydial or viral swabs, the patient needs to understand what we have done, and also be aware of the implications of a positive test. The patient needs to understand that some infections may be present for years, and do not imply that a partner has had another recent sexual partner.

It is also important that clinicians know their tests, as some may come up with false positives, and require confirmation. Chlamydia, in particular, has several different diagnostic tests available, with relative problems of false positives, false negatives or higher costs. Some tests even vary considerably in the hands of different laboratories. Finding out about the test that you use is a part of the process of adequately advising your patient. GUM clinics will confirm diagnoses if there is uncertainity.

case study

Emma and Jake had been together 3 years. They were worried about their baby Adam's sticky eye, and took him to see their GP when Adam was six weeks old. The GP did both an ordinary and a chlamydial swab, and explained that if they were both clear, it was likely to be a blocked duct.

When the chlamydial culture came back positive, the GP found herself in deep water, because she had not prepared the ground at the time of doing the test. Whilst trying to explain why all three of them would need treatment, it became clear that Emma thought she and Jake's relationship was mutually a first and monogamous one. The couple left, appearing tense and confused. Jake's brief relationship with someone else a year before was revealed to Emma that evening. Emma was very distressed, and there was a considerable strain on the relationship for some time.

The GP felt she could have handled the whole thing with considerably more caution, and perhaps made the outcome a little more easy to handle by giving more information when the swab was taken. Jake would then have had time to consider the information, and handle his disclosure under slightly less pressure.

Consent and insurance medical reports

There is evidence that only about half of patients who have applied for life insurance were aware that they have signed consent for a medical report to be completed about them by their GP[15]. Half the patients imagined that their doctor would protect their interests, withholding information that was sensitive. It is therefore questionable whether the consent usually obtained is in fact informed consent.

Some practices avoid this problem by seeking consent with a simply worded letter to the patient, pointing out that they should see the doctor concerned if they have any queries. Impetus is added if it is also pointed out that the report will not be completed until consent has been received.

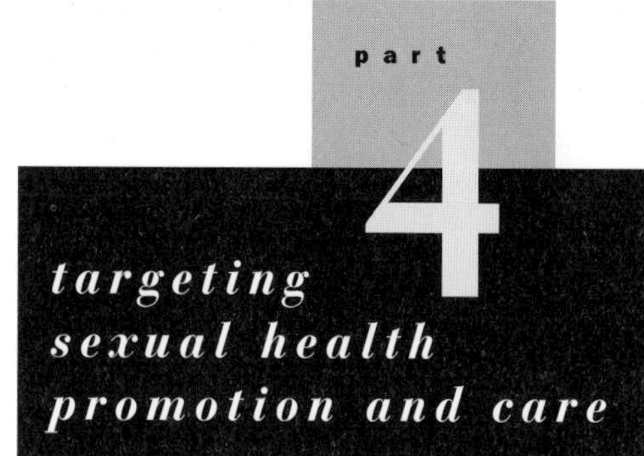

part 4 *targeting sexual health promotion and care*

Even those most enthusiastic about sexual health promotion need to make decisions about which patients to target, and when. As with much of our work, pressures of time may limit what we can do. For this reason it is worth identifying patients or clinical contexts which will be prioritised for sexual health work. This is likely to have a knock-on effect, as the more experience staff have of sexual health work, the easier it is to raise the subject in varied clinical contexts.

Effective, opportunistic sexual health promotion may involve raising the topic of sexual health in a way that may seem 'out of the blue' to the patient (for example, when they come for travel advice or a new patient check). Approaches to introducing the topic of sexual health are discussed on pages 20–31.

Each team will need to consider which approaches to sexual health promotion seem most pertinent to the patients they serve.

Targeting an age group

Many practices choose to prioritise the under 25s, although sexually transmitted infections and unintended pregnancies are not rare in those older than this. Some practices run young people's clinics aimed at teenagers which deal with sexual health issues.

Maximise opportunities to work with men

Men consult less frequently than women in primary care, and for this reason clinical staff should consider when they could do sexual health promotion. A good opportunity is when they come for travel advice. Another possibility is in new patient checks, or entirely opportunistically when men are consulting for other reasons (if time allows). Practice nurses can play a key role here.

Contraceptive services

Sexual health promotion should be considered an integral part of contraceptive provision, as a minimum at the first consultation. Our 'pill starting' clinical routines should be reviewed to ensure that competent histories are being taken in order to assess the woman's risk of acquiring STIs. She can then be advised accordingly about condom use. Such an assessment is also imperative for women considering the use of intrauterine contraceptive devices or long acting progestogen contraception by injection or implant. Similarly women who choose barrier methods should be advised about emergency contraception in case they failed to use them or had a problem with them.

Cervical screening

When conducting a smear there is often time to take a sexual history and do some sexual health promotion work. This groundwork may smooth the way in case an STI is identified on the smear test. In some practices the history then helps inform a decision on whether to screen for chlamydia at the same time as taking a smear. The identification of infections on a smear result should trigger an appropriate response from clinicians, including consideration of treatment, contacts, the possibility of other infections co-existing, and finally sexual health promotion so the woman understands how to avoid further infections. GUM clinic referral will often be appropriate.

Condom distribution

Many practices are now involved in condom distribution. These practices should consider the following points:

- Do they ensure that patients have the correct information and teaching to use condoms safely? Where are male condom demonstrators kept, and how often are they used?
- How accessible are condoms in the practice – where are they kept? Who is giving them out?
- Are appropriate measures in place to ensure those who practice anal intercourse obtain extra-strong condoms and lubricant?
- Are bags available to put condoms in when they are being given out?
- Are systems in place to allow easy and confidential access to condoms for patients who are regular users, and know which type they need? Some practices give a discreet card to patients which they can give to the receptionist. The card code indicates condom type needed.
- Are heterosexual couples using condoms informed about emergency contraception?

Travel advice

Studies conducted in genitourinary medicine clincs show international travellers may be at considerable risk of acquiring sexually transmitted infections[16,17]. In primary care, we may well see these patients before departure. An assessment should be made of the likelihood of this risk through the history, in order to target advice and information. Holidays may be viewed by the patient as as an opportunity to find new sexual partners, or to buy sex. Both in continental Europe and elsewhere there are many holiday destinations where the prevalence of HIV is substantially greater that in the UK. Patients should also be informed that it is prudent to take supplies of appropriate condoms, and they should have the Kitemark or CE mark of quality pointed out to them. It may be an opportunity to check immunity or immunise patients against hepatitis B.

New patient checks

These checks provide an excellent opportunity for sexual health promotion, most obviously with women. Such checks often include questions about smears and contraception, and thus it is relatively easy to move into other aspects of sexual health. For men the transition may seem harder, but confidence soon comes with familiarity with such work (see *Examples of patient check forms for women and men,* pages 47–48).

How some practices have improved their sexual health service

Below are experiences drawn from different practices which have tried to improve sexual health promotion and care. Each of the teams has learnt to identify and respond to the needs of the population for whom they care.

case study

One practice changed its new patient check forms to have one for men and one for women – so all the checks ended by doing some sexual history taking and sexual health promotion. Men and women were advised about condom availability and emergency contraception, otherwise they differed. According to the practice nurse: 'Particularly the young men seem to appreciate being given an opportunity to discuss sexual health. They often have real concerns and questions to ask. We seem to have changed the atmosphere a bit, and we have a few young men who come here regularly for condoms.'

case study

A practice serves an urban area with a large Asian population. One of the practice nurses came across this story. A young man was being encouraged to use prostitutes on a trip to Delhi, in order to gain sexual experience. It was thought by his (older) adviser that Delhi sex workers were 'safe' – unlike those in the UK, who, it was considered might 'have AIDS'. This event triggered the practice to develop an approach that considered the sexual health promotion needs of travellers to the Indian subcontinent. The practice nurse also contacted a link worker in the local health promotion unit for advice on the development of a culturally appropriate information campaign on HIV risks.

case study

Lisa is a nurse in a practice which has quite a large number of intravenous drug users. A significant number of these are HIV positive. 'It makes little sense to talk about condoms and safer sex without thinking about the drug side of things. Our practice had to come up with an approach that would think about safe needle use as well as safer sex. We also try to be aware that people may sell sex in order to pay for their drugs. Other things come up – like discussions about how drugs or alcohol cloud intentions to use condoms. And we like to think we're red hot on hep B immunisation!'

case study

Melanie is a GP in a practice in a small town in a rural area. 'I was interested in chlamydia, because I'd been trained in a big city. I thought it wouldn't be relevant here, but then I found out that our local teenage pregnancy rates were pretty high. Together with the practice nurse we had a real drive to improve contraception provision for young people, and we started to look for chlamydia more. As we came across quite a few cases, we decided to do a proper screening study – taking swabs from all women under 25 who came for a pelvic examination. We were shocked to find a rate of about 6 per cent. All the clinical staff are right up to speed now. We've even done our own info sheet on chlamydia aimed at young people. It's so hard to get the message across that it doesn't necessarily have symptoms, yet can do so much harm.'

Figure 1: Example of patient registration form

Welcome
Name ______
Address ______
______
______
Preferred title ______
Date of Birth ______
Tel no ______
Computer no. ______

Last GP:
Name ______
Address ______
______
______

Employment status
Full-time/Part-time/Unemployed
Job/last job:
______
How would you describe your ethnic group?
______
Health check appointment given YES/NO

Please read our practice leaflet. It contains useful information. Please attend your health check. It is important for your care!

Figure 2: Example of patient check form for women

Name **Computer number**
Domestic status/Household
Children: names and date of birth

Health check date

Height	Urine	Last tetanus
Weight	Blood pressure	Last polio
Body mass index		Daily tobacco
Diet:	Exercise:	Weekly alcohol

Current medication: Record certainties on computer –
1
2
3
4
5

Allergies: Record on folder/computer
1
2

Past medical history: Record certainties on summary/computer

Family history – Check epilepsy, CVS, diabetes, glaucoma, cancer and asthma

	Age	Health	Cause of death	Age at death
Mother				
Father				
Brother(s)				
Sister(s)				

Sexual health – Women Please write years*

PREGNANCIES	Live birth*	Miscarriage*	TOP* Still birth*
HYSTERECTOMY Yes/No	Reason:	MAMMOGRAM*	Breast awareness
LAST CERVICAL SMEAR Date:	Place:	Past abnormality?	

Need of CONTRACEPTION? if so, what used? FP 1001 needed? YES/NO
Need of CONDOMS YES/NO Supply from here? (Check able to use, appropriate type) YES/NO
Aware of availability of EMERGENCY CONTRACEPTION and appropriate use / how to access
Raised by nurse or doctor? Assess risk STIs/safer sex Raised? – YES/NO
Drug use Raised? YES/NO
use 'open door' statement if NO

Figure 3: Example of patient check form for men

Name **Computer number**

Domestic status/Household

Children: names and DOB

Health check date

Height	Urine	Last tetanus
Weight	BP	Last polio
BMI		Daily tobacco
Diet:	Exercise:	Weekly alcohol

Current medication: Record certainties on computer –

1
2
3
4
5
6

Allergies: Record on folder/computer

1
2

Past medical history: Record certainties on summary/computer

Family history – Check epilepsy, CVS, diabetes, glaucoma, cancer and asthma

	Age	Health	Cause of death	Age at death
Mother				
Father				
Brother(s)				
Sister(s)				

Sexual health – Men

Need of CONDOMS? Supply from here? (Check able to use, appropriate type given) YES/NO

Aware of availability of emergency contraception and appropriate use?

PROSTATE AWARENESS: TESTICULAR SELF EXAMINATION:

Raised by nurse or doctor? Assess risk STIs/safer sex Raised? – YES/NO

Drug use Raised? YES/NO

use 'open door'statement if NO?

part 5

key messages

- GPs and practice nurses need to be aware that two or more of the clinical areas of sexual health (contraception, psychosexual issues and STIs) may inter-relate in individual patients with important clinical consequences
- The quality of the clinical care you provide in sexual health work will be profoundly influenced by whether – and how – you ask key questions of your patients
- Asking intimate questions in a considered and caring way will be found to become easier and rewarding with time. Start to reflect on your practice now!
- Many significant psychological or sexual health problems may remain invisible if clinical practice is not conducted in a way that is seen to be open and accepting by important groups (for example young people, those in same-sex relationships and older patients)
- Never initiate provision of a non-barrier contraceptive without a careful assessment of the need for additional barrier contraception. Never assume someone who has no need for contraception has no need for protection from STIs
- Educators hold our future: sexual history skills are a basic clinical skill for GPs and practice nurses, but currently are rarely taught

part 6

further reading

- ***Women' s sexual health***
  Andrews G (ed)
  Balliere Tindall, 1997
- ***Blocks and freedoms in sexual life***
  Skrine R
  Radcliffe Medical Press, 1997
- ***Sexual history taking in general practice***
  Jewitt C
  The HIV Project, London, 1995
- ***Confidentiality and people under 16***
  BMA, Brook, GMSC, FPA, HEA and RCGP, joint guidance, 1993.
- ***Discussing sex***
  Louis Levy
  Lambeth, Southwark and Lewisham HA, 1997

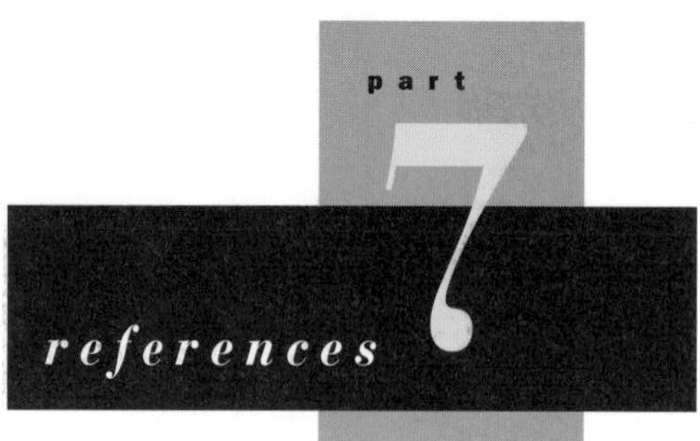

1 'Who goes to sexually transmitted disease clinics? Results from a national population survey' Johnson AM, Wadsworth J and Wellings K, et al, ***Genitourinary Medicine, 72***, 1996, 197-202

2 'Do teenagers consult general practitioners for contraceptive advice?' Seamark CJ and Pereira Gray DJ, ***British Journal of Family Planning, 21***, 1995, 50-51

3 'STD awareness today' Bleker OP, ***Genitourinary Medicine, 72***, 1996, 440-442

4 ***Confidentiality and people under 16***, BMA, Brook, FPA GMSC, HEA, and RCGP, joint guidance 1993

5 'Domestic violence and pregnancy' editorial, Mezey GC and Bewley S, ***British Medical Journal, 314***, 1997, 1295

6 'Domestic violence: a hidden problem for general practice,' Richardson J and Feder G, ***British Journal of General Practice, 46,*** 1996, 239-42

7 'A case-controlled study of the sexual health needs of lesbians,' Skinner CJ, Stokes J and Kirlew Y et al, ***Genitourinary Medicine, 72***, 1996, 277-280

8 ***Guidelines for pre-test discussion on HIV testing***, Department of Health, 1996

9 ***Sexual health and family planning services in general practice,*** FPA, 1993

10 General Medical Council guidelines, 'Duties of a doctor' series. 'You must not allow your views about a patient's lifestyle, sexuality, (or) age....to prejudice the treatment you give or arrange' (from ***'Good Medical Practice'*** booklet, 1995). Other booklets deal with HIV and AIDS and with confidentiality

11 ***The nursing care of lesbians and gay men***, Royal College of Nurses statement RCN, 1994

12 ***Family planning and pregnancy counselling projects for young people***, Allen I, Policy Studies Institute, 1991

13 'Survey of HIV patients views on confidentiality and non-discrimination policies in general practice' Shaw M, Tomlinson D and Higginson I, ***British Medical Journal***, ***312***, 1996, 1463-64

14 'Perceptions of general practice among homosexual men,' Fitzpatrick R, Dawson J and Boulton M, et al, ***British Journal of General Practice***, ***44***, 1994, 80-82

15 'How informed is patients' consent to release of medical information to insurance companies?' Lorge RE ***British Medical Journal, 298,*** 1989, 1495-6

16 'Risk behaviour and STD acquisition in genitourinary clinic attenders who have travelled' Hawkes S, Hart GJ, and Bletsoe E, et al, ***Genitourinary Medicine, 71***, 1995, 351-354

25 'Sexual behaviour in travellers abroad attending an inner-city genitourinary medicine clinic,' Mendelsohn R, Astle L and Mann M, et al, ***Genitourinary Medicine***, ***72***, 1996, 43-46

Acknowledgements

My thanks go to Sarah Madge and Riva Miller (for the *HIV testing...in general practice* box) and to Lis Hughes, for everything.

Philippa Matthews

Anne Damerell

Catti Moss

chapter three

confidentiality

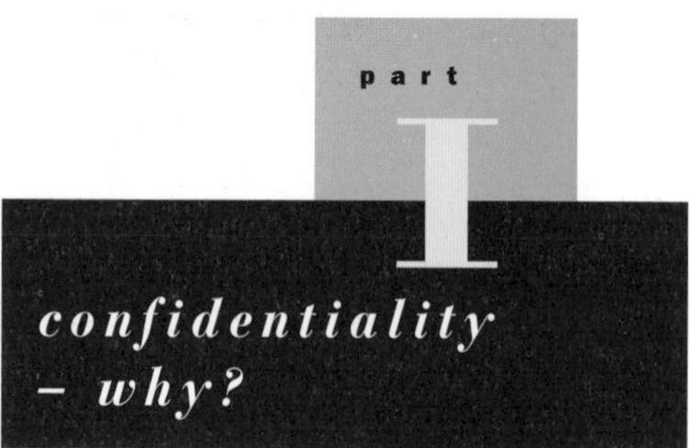

confidentiality – why?

In the same way that patients can choose what they tell us about themselves, they should have the right to decide how far information about them is shared with others. In practical terms, confidentiality is the basis of the relationship of trust between patient and doctor (or any health professional), as good medical practice depends on patients being able to talk freely about any aspect of their health.

Legislation

Medical confidentiality is not protected by statute like that of the lawyer, but is a common law duty, which will be enforced by professional bodies and by the courts[1]. There is little legislation about medical confidentiality, and individual judgments in cases brought before the courts form the basis of the legal situation.

- The Data Protection Act introduced controls over data held on computer, and first gave patients access to their computer record
- The Access to Health Records Act 1990 gave patients the right to see their written medical records, though, as it was not retrospective, the rights do not extend to records before 1991

The practical necessity of confidentiality, and its moral and legal rights, are brought into sharp focus when considering issues of sexual health. There is legislation specific to sexual and reproductive issues which enhances the rights and duties of confidentiality in these circumstances.

- The Human Fertilisation and Embryology (Disclosure of Information) Act 1992 put limits on disclosure on a need to know basis with the patient's consent.
- The Gillick judgment in 1985 established the right of under-age girls to contraception without the consent or knowledge of parents. It made clear that minors who are able fully to understand what is proposed and have sufficient discretion to make a wise choice in their best interests are competent to consent to medical treatment regardless of age[2,3].
- The Children Act 1989 confirmed the right of minors to refuse examination or assessment. It emphasised the role of children and young people in decision-making and encouraged doctors to develop techniques for consulting them.[4]
- The NHS (Venereal Disease) Regulations SI(74)29 imposed a statutory obligation on health authorities, (though not on GPs), to prevent the identification of individuals who have been treated for any sexually transmitted infection. These regulations are held to apply to all cases of HIV infection, however acquired[5]

Trust

Patients' need for privacy and confidentiality is at its greatest in sexual health. If they do not feel confident that information about them will be secure, they will not reveal it, or will not come for help at all. The consequences may be unwanted pregnancy, illegal abortion, untreated disease, and unnecessary misery and distress. A survey[6] of 662 HIV positive patients in 1993–4 showed that only 58 per cent of them were registered with a GP who knew their diagnosis. Good practice must be confidential, and must be seen and believed to be confidential by the people who matter – our patients. Section 2 offers some ideas on how to achieve these ends.

Minors
The duty of confidentiality owed to a person under 16 is as great as that owed to any other person. Regardless of whether or not the requested treatment is given, the confidentiality of the consultation should still be respected, unless there are convincing reasons to the contrary[7].

There are special problems for young people, particularly minors. In 1993, joint guidance on confidentiality and people under 16 was published by the British Medical Association (BMA), the Royal College of General Practitioners (RCGP), the Family Planning Association (FPA), the General Medical Services Committee (GMSC), the Health Education Authority (HEA) and Brook Advisory Centres[5]. This states clearly that any competent young person, regardless of age, can independently seek medical advice and give valid consent to medical treatment (see box). Despite this, a survey of 1869 young people aged 12–19 in 1995 by Northamptonshire Multidiscipline Audit Advisory Group showed that 58 per cent of them thought that their parents would hear about it if they visited the doctor[8]. To change this belief may be the most important task for primary care to tackle in order to improve sexual health services for this age group.

Exceptions

Sometimes the law requires us to disclose confidential information, and in extremely rare cases, we may need to do so in a patients' interests. We must be prepared to explain and justify our decisions if this happens. Part 3 (page 57) gives some examples of such cases.

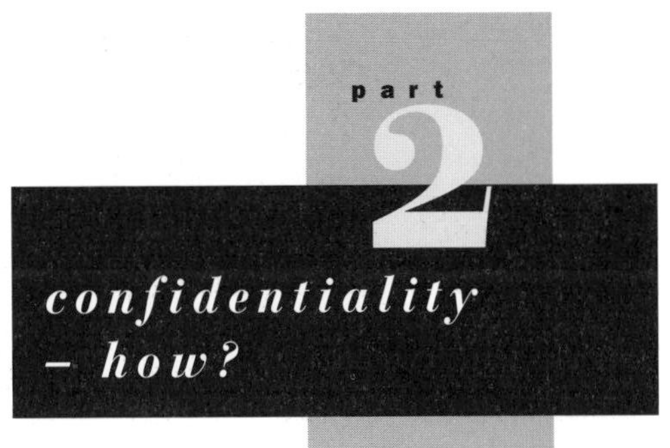

part 2 confidentiality – how?

Raise the issue

Everyone who works in the practice, including doctors and nurses, must fully understand and respect the need for confidentiality, while working in the practice, and subsequently. Everyone should be familiar with the important basic guidelines, such as the General Medical Council (GMC) booklet on confidentiality[9]. Confidentiality issues should be discussed, not only when staff are beginning their job, but in a regular and recurring way, with the whole team. Training must keep up with changing working conditions: for example, bringing up a patient's record on a computer screen without good reason feels less like a breach of privacy than opening a drawer, getting out the patient's folder and reading it, but the actions are morally and practically equivalent.

example

Nurse: *'She's gone into hospital, she's on Ward 17'.*
This information may not be innocuous if Ward 17 treats patients with AIDS, or is the ward for patients having terminations.

Make receptionists doubly aware

In most GP practices, receptionists have to easy access to medical records because they are the people who get the notes out for surgeries etc, and type in test results and other information. The number of people with such access is increased if the surgery has many part-time clerical staff, or a frequent turnover of staff, or if agency staff are brought in to bring records up to date. Patients may not be aware how much access receptionists have to information about them, and may not find this acceptable. In the survey[6] already mentioned, 70 per cent of the patients objected to receptionists knowing their diagnosis – over 20 per cent more than for any other staff group. At the National Association for Patient Participation in May 1996 members expressed concern that medical histories were known to large numbers of clerical staff. Carman and Britten[10] found that patients object more to their records being seen by staff in general practice than by relatively anonymous hospital staff.

example

Patient at reception:
'I've come for my test results'
Receptionist:
'What test was that dear?'
Three people in the queue prick up their ears.

Control information given to other groups
Many groups of staff, such as therapists, counsellors, and health visitors, should only give and receive information on a need-to-know basis. The House of Commons Social Services Committee said (re problems with AIDS, 1987) that in practice 'there should be a very strict need-to-know policy: those involved in the direct care of a person must be told, but there is no need for everyone involved in the care to be told the exact diagnosis[11]. All staff who come in contact with patients should already be observing strict hygiene, and precautions as if every patient were HIV positive. The sharing of identifiable information for the convenience or interests of health workers or administrators cannot be justified[12]. The whole primary health care team should be aware of the practice policy, and the reasons for it.

Ask patients about records
If patients give you sensitive information, before writing it in the notes, ask them how far it may be shared within the multidisciplinary team[9]. Always find out what information they regard as confidential, as one person's mortifying secret may be another's commonplace. Consider whether the information should be recorded in the notes at all, and how to record it if it is needed. If the patient moves and changes doctor, their future GP may have very different ideas about what is suitable to put in an insurance or employment report. The RCGP, in its leaflet *You and your GP during the day* (1997), advises patients that 'you can discuss with your GP what you would like put in your records and whether there is anything which you want to be kept private between the two of you'. Remember to tell patients that they may have to remind you about non-recorded information at subsequent consultations.

The following are examples of facts which *may* not need to be recorded in the notes:

- sexual orientation
- transsexualism
- names of sexual partners
- a previous abortion
- asymptomatic HIV status
- that a child has been conceived by donor insemination
- attendance at a GUM clinic
- requests for contraception – in particular from minors, but older single women may also regard this as an extremely private matter. (A prescription for the pill should be recorded, but the reason need not)

Make premises suitable
Confidentiality may depend on the layout of the building. Consulting rooms should be soundproofed and not sited directly off the waiting room. Patients in the waiting room should not be able to hear what is said at the reception counter, and patients at the reception counter should not be able to hear staff talking on the telephone. It is not possible to change bricks and mortar easily or quickly, but by working out where the problems are, it may be possible to solve them by other means, eg canned music, white noise, or changing the use of telephones.

example

Receptionist on telephone:
'Ah Miss Brown we've had the result and you're not pregnant'
But the caller was actually Mrs Brown who sounds like her daughter on the telephone

Practice telephone discretion

All staff in reception should be in the habit of discretion at all times, to avoid overhearing by people waiting to be seen. This involves never using names of patients or saying anything that might identify the patient. Listeners at the surgery end may be no wiser, if the name is a common one, but a glance at the telephone directory will confirm that not many of us are in fact called Smith, Brown or Patel. Many people have names which only occur a few times in each district; such people are instantly identifiable by any mention of their name. Repeating addresses back should also be avoided.

Ensure private information reaches the right ears

It is impossible to guarantee that information given out by telephone or letter will reach the intended recipient and nobody else. The best way to ensure that no third party has access to information is to give it in the privacy of the consulting room. Even giving the message that the patient should go and see the doctor may break confidentiality, so it is important to make firm arrangements for results at the time of arranging the tests.

Keep notes in the right place

Make sure that there is no public access to any area where records are kept, and equally that records are not accessible in any public area, such as a treatment room which takes two or more patients at the same time. Make sure that notes are kept secure when out visiting.

Consider the problems that arise from research and audit

Many research projects involve extracting information from patient notes, and in these cases the patients may not be informed of this. Very often a researcher from outside the practice will be given the run of the files, in order to extract the information needed. This breaches confidentiality, and many patients would be extremely unhappy about it. Audit causes few problems when contained within the practice, but the trend towards multi-practice collaborative audits means that sometimes outsiders are given access to the notes for these.

Make special arrangements if you are a training practice

Training practices are required to be visited and assessed at regular intervals. The teams that visit are usually doctors, but include practice managers in at least one region. The visitors will need to look at notes in the course of the assessment. Patients should be informed that this happens, by a notice in the surgery, and a paragraph in the surgery brochure and news sheet. Video recordings of surgery consultations are now almost mandatory during registrar training. Fortunately, a high standard of informed, written consent is expected. However, problems can arise if videos are not wiped clean after they are finished with, or if they are stored insecurely. If consent for a video specifies one use or audience, fresh consent from the patient must be sought if a new use is planned, or if it will be shown to a wider audience.

Keep computer hardware secure

Most practices have virtually no protection for the increasing amount of data on computers. Already surgeries are a frequent target for computer thieves, who usually steal the main part of the computer (with the hard disk). At the moment the computer is usually cannibalised for the chip, and the rest discarded, but it will not be long before someone sees the possibility of all that health information. The Data Protection Registrar requires doctors to protect computers and software from theft from surgery premises and cars. The current recommendation is for steel cages around main computers.

Keep computer software secure

While computers stand alone in surgeries they are relatively safe from hackers, but as modems are connected they become at risk. As the NHS develops networks and systems for the electronic transfer of letters and test results, this problem must be dealt with effectively. On a more practical level, ensure that the passwords you use are not too obvious and make sure that all staff shut down the computer properly when they leave.

example

A GP's husband, who was called in to sort out a problem, took less than 2 minutes to guess the passwords and start up the system despite having no previous knowledge of it.

Keep fax security

Only send faxes with identifiable information when the receiving machine is known to be secure – in and out of working hours.

Shred

Always shred all redundant paper records before disposal. Murphy's Law states that if you do not meticulously observe this rule, some records will leap from a bursting black bag on to the front page of the local newspaper.

example

The schoolgirl who finds her teacher in the next chair in the family planning clinic queue may be embarrassed but what happens when her mother arrives for the weight watchers' club which assembles nearby?

Organise for privacy and anonymity

The advantages of confidentiality afforded by family planning clinics may be lost if the clinic patients are identifiable as a group. If the queue sits in a designated area, or if patients are called by name from a common waiting area, by an identifiable clinician, the nature of their problem is publicised. Effective appointments systems should be in use to minimise the number of patients waiting together, and they should wait out of sight of other patients. Combined well-woman and family planning clinics convey less specific messages to outsiders and may therefore be more acceptable to users.

example

A GUM clinic flourished in an obscure building until it was rationalised into a local community hospital and forced to conform to its standard procedure whereby patients for several clinics shared the same waiting area, and were called by name from it, to an identifiable room. Attendances dropped and the clinic closed.

Consider language and cultural needs

Many women who speak little English take a male relative with them to the doctor to interpret for them. In areas of sexual health this may infringe their confidentiality, and make it difficult to meet their needs. If there are people in this position in your practice, it may be possible to arrange for them to come with an independent interpreter, or a patient advocate.

Meet your community's special needs

It may be particularly difficult to maintain confidentiality in small communities, where everyone knows everyone else. This may not only be in small towns, but in tightly-knit groups in inner-cities. In some rural areas there is no way for adolescents without transport to use anonymous family planning clinics, and the surgery may appear to be full of their parents' friends. In a small town presenting a prescription at the pharmacy may feel very public. With careful and ingenious thought you may find acceptable local solutions. There are many quirks in the rules that may help. (For instance, it is possible to sign someone on as a 'contraceptive only' patient.)

Be seen to be confidential

Consider agreeing your position on

confidentiality within the practice, and writing a statement to put in practice leaflets and charters, and on posters in the surgery. As well as generalities, it may be useful to mention specific local issues. However, word your statement carefully, to avoid making a totally open-ended promise that might not be possible to keep in the very unusual cases where disclosure may be necessary.

AN EXAMPLE STATEMENT OF CONFIDENTIALITY COULD BE

'We have strict rules about confidentiality which apply to all our staff. We are especially careful that family members should not be able to learn things about each other unless consent has been given by the patient concerned. If you have worries about confidentiality please feel free to discuss it with our doctors or nurses.'

Additions could be:

'If you would like a discussion left off your record just mention this to the doctor at the start of your appointment.'

'If you would like to see our practice confidentiality policy please contact our practice manager.'

Most disclosure of personal information is done with the patient's consent, real or assumed. The rare instances of disclosure without consent get a disproportionate amount of thought and public attention, but the problems are as real and important in the areas where we take things for granted.

Sharing information within the primary health care team

Effective teamwork in general practice is not possible without sharing patient information. Most of us assume that this has the consent of patients, and in practice there are rarely problems. Surveys of what patients think[6,10] reveal that we may be wrong in this assumption. In doubtful or sensitive situations, such consent should be explicitly sought[9], and special arrangements made.

External requests for information

We are increasingly bombarded with requests for information about patients, from social service departments, lawyers, employers, and insurance companies. The cardinal principle in dealing with these is to speak to the patient and obtain informed consent before any disclosure. Fraudulent attempts to obtain information are made, eg using solicitor's headed paper, and a forged permission to release information. We are rarely familiar with our patients' signatures. By contacting the patient fraud will be exposed, and it is possible to confirm the precise nature of the information that should be given, and make arrangements for seeing the report, if that is desired.

case study

One inner city practice serves a population with a high number of gay and bisexual men. As the team made efforts to address the health needs of this group of patients, they began to be concerned about the implications of a record of sexuality in the notes. Whilst the practice had a watertight policy on the avoidance of vague questions in insurance questionnaires, future GPs of the patients may not have the same approach. After much discussion, the team reluctantly agreed that the only safe option was not to record sexuality at all, unless patients were fully informed and emphatic that they wished a record to be kept. Team members would explain this policy to new patients, who were encouraged to mention their sexuality in future consultations if they felt it was relevant. The system works reasonably well and at least demonstrates to concerned gay patients that their needs have been carefully considered by the team.

Life insurance

People wanting life insurance, mortgages, etc. have to sign a form in which they consent to the divulging of any information held by the GP in their records. This can hardly be described as free or informed consent, especially as many people never realise exactly what they have agreed to. Disclosure of confidential information about a patient in these circumstances is a breach of the trust between doctor and patient, and fear of such disclosure may lead patients to conceal sensitive information such as HIV status from us. The RCGP recommended in 1991 that doctors should not answer lifestyle questions on such forms. The BMA agrees, and states also that doctors should not agree to speculate on the patient's risk of death or disease[2]. Insurance companies will usually accept forms with contentious questions left blank or marked 'lifestyle question – not applicable', but it is difficult to remember not to fill in the spaces. A rubber stamp saying 'This practice does not answer lifestyle questions, in line with BMA guidance', is not only easier to use, but seems to be more acceptable to insurance companies. It is arguable[14] that GPs should refuse to supply any information to insurance companies. The company would then have to arrange for the patient to be medically examined by another doctor, not the usual GP. In this way patients would regain responsibility for health information supplied to outside bodies.

Insurance medical reports...in practice

- **The UK is the only country in which insurance companies can access comprehensive medical information from personal medical attendants**
- **Half of patients are unaware they have given consent to have a medical report done**
- **Half of patients think their doctor will withold information to protect their confidentiality**
- **GPs may therefore wish to take steps to gain informed consent before completing a form**
- **Doctors should not answer 'lifestyle' questions. Their knowledge of their patients' HIV risk may be poor. Sexuality should never be taken as a proxy for risk**
- **A common response used by GPs to answer lifestyle questions is 'please refer question to patient'**
- **BMA recommendations appear likely to change. They will indicate that a history of a sexually transmitted infection should not be disclosed unless the infection has ongoing clinical implications**
- **All clinical workers in a practice should understand the implications of the written record, should it follow the patient to a GP with a discriminatory or ill-considered approach to completing insurance medical reports**

Reports to employers

The same principles apply to pre-employment reports and medicals. Job discrimination based on HIV status cannot be justified by the risk of transmission.

Patients who cannot consent

Insurance companies sometimes seek medical information about a patient who has died, when settling claims on the policy. BMA guidance that doctors should not issue such 'duration certificates' had to be reviewed when the Access to Health Records Act 1990 gave a legal right of access to people with a claim related to the death. However, confidentiality after the patient's death is still the expected norm; and legally doctors should still refuse to disclose information provided by the patient in the expectation that it would remain confidential. Wherever possible, doctors should advise patients in advance to specify any sensitive matters which should not be disclosed after death[15].

Breaking confidentiality

Total confidentiality is not always in the patient's or public interest. The guidance of bodies such as the GMC, GMSC and Royal College of Nursing (RCN) is that there are circumstances where information should be revealed, even if patients do not consent[11]. Some areas related to sexual health where this may happen are discussed below. All are unusual, none are totally clear cut.

Child sexual abuse

This is an area which can cause the greatest difficulty. Most districts have explicit guidelines for all relevant professionals, that allow no flexibility, and that state that social services should be informed automatically, in all cases, with or without the consent of the patient. Social services consider that people are children up to the age of 18. If you only suspect that a young patient is being sexually abused or exploited, you should assess the evidence carefully, remembering the devastating effects on the family of a false allegation of sexual abuse. There would have to be clear evidence both that abuse was taking place, and that disclosure would protect a child in danger, before breaching confidentiality here. If a child reveals sexual abuse, the situation is more clear cut. Most children agree that their troubles should not be kept secret, and are extremely relieved that action will be taken. If a child is not happy for you to tell anyone else, the first thing to consider is whether they are able to understand the implications of their decision. Quite young children can make an informed judgement, and in general their confidence should be kept, while encouraging them to think about changing the decision in the future. However, there may be an immediate serious risk of harm, either to the child or to another person (eg a sibling) and here informing social services may be in their best interests[16]. Occasionally there is a real conflict of interest between a child who has revealed abuse, and other children who are at risk. In the end, the principal concern must be the welfare of the child.

Crime

Sexual health consultations may be times when patients unburden themselves of painful secrets, and they may tell us about crimes committed either by them or to them. Rape, assault, incest, infanticide or other crimes may be revealed. The common law consensus is that doctors have a duty to report 'serious crime' that overrides patient confidentiality. There is no consensus on where the boundary between 'serious' and 'ordinary' crime lies. In general, confidentiality should be respected, unless the health or safety of others will be endangered by keeping silent. The cases of Beverly Allitt and Amanda Jenkinson (both nurses who endangered the health of patients in their care, while suffering from mental illness that was not revealed to their employers) have opened a new debate, and more precise guidelines may very well result.

HIV infection

An HIV positive person who cannot be persuaded to inform or to protect a partner or partners poses problems which have no easy answers. The GMC's guidance[9] is that 'there are grounds for disclosure only when there is a serious and identifiable risk to a specific individual, who, if not so informed, would be exposed to infection'. If you consider breaching confidentiality here, the onus lies with you to demonstrate not only that it would be morally justified, but also that it is likely to achieve its intended purpose. Disclosure may not greatly reduce the risk to the patient's contacts if they have many sexual partners or share needles. More people may be infected in the end if the patient loses faith in, and contact with, doctors. On the other hand, Gillett[17] gives the example of a man who refuses to reveal his HIV status to his wife, with the result that they both die and their children are orphaned. He says 'it seems just plain wrong for the doctor to sit back and allow her to fall victim to a fatal disease because of the wish of her husband'. It is possible that this will some day be tested in the courts by a relative who believes that a doctor's inaction has caused the death of a loved one.

It is also possible that an indignant partner may react to disclosure by publicising the HIV status of the patient, who may then face hostility and prejudice, and the loss of friends, job, or housing. Fear and ignorance about the risks of HIV transmission are still widespread, though we may hope that the situation has improved since 1986, when an ambulance crew burnt their uniforms after taking an injured HIV positive person to hospital[18].

Decision-making

There are many other examples of where it may be necessary to breach confidentiality, not all related to sexual health. All are unusual and difficult situations. Because these are outside our normal experience, partners and colleagues are unlikely to be able to give informed advice. Fortunately, the medical defence organisations will offer free immediate and confidential advice over the telephone. If the patient's name is omitted, privacy will be preserved. It may be possible to get two independent expert views if partners have different defence organisations. Alternatively, the BMA could be approached directly for advice. Having consulted expert outsiders, the decision must be taken personally, and may still not be easy. It may be helpful to consider ethical principles in balancing the conflicting interests. This involves identifying the possible courses of action, and then considering the effects of each separately, under the headings of:

- beneficence (the amount of good that would be done)
- maleficence (the amount of harm that would be done)
- patient autonomy (how the patients rights will be respected)
- social justice (how society and others are protected)

Whatever your decision, this would mean that if it was questioned you could show your reasoning in a clear and acceptable way.

part 4 key messages

- Medical confidentiality is a common law duty, and not directly protected by legislation
- Groups of patients who feel vulnerable have expressed concerns about GP confidentiality
- We owe a duty of confidentiality to all patients, whatever their age or condition
- The need for privacy is at its greatest in sexual health
- Make confidentiality an important issue for the whole team
- Record only the information that you need, and negotiate about sensitive items
- Keep records, whether paper, computer or tape in a secure fashion
- Prevent people from overhearing information
- Organise surgeries and clinics for privacy and anonymity
- Make special arrangements for the community's special needs
- Patients may not be happy for information to be shared within the primary health care team
- Always check consent before revealing information
- Not all lawyers letters or medical report forms are genuine
- In sexual abuse, local guidelines may be prescriptive
- Ask for advice before breaking confidence.
- Be prepared to justify in detail any breach of confidence

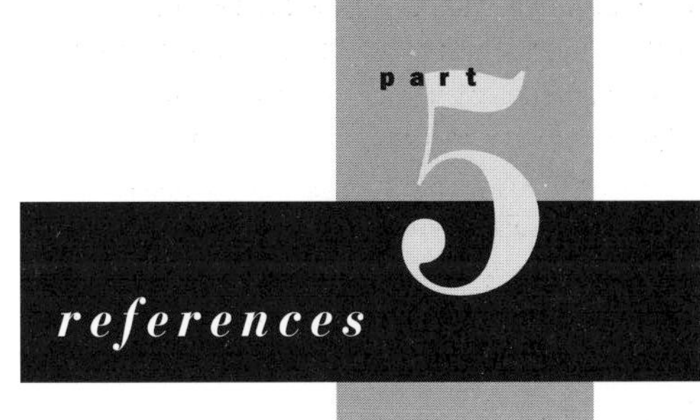

part 5 references

1 ***Rights and responsibilities of doctors – A guide to the law as it affects doctors***, BMA, 1992, 36

2 ***Medical ethics today: its practice and philosophy***, BMA, 1993, 72-81

3 ***Doctors' decisions: ethical conflicts in medical practice***, Dunstan GR and Shinebourne EA (eds), Oxford University Press, 1989, 86-87

4 See ref 2 above, page 73

5 See ref 1 above, page 53

6 'Survey of HIV patients' views on confidentiality and non-discrimination policies in general practice', Shaw M, Tomlinson D and Higginson I, ***British Medical Journal, 312***, 1996, 1463-64

7 ***Confidentiality and people under 16***, BMA, Brook, FPA, GMSC, HEA and RCGP, Joint guidance, 1993

8 ***Sexual health services for young people: a county-wide audit***, Hunt J, Northants MAAG, 1995

9 'Confidentiality', ***Duties of a doctor***, GMC, 1995

10 'Confidentiality of medical records: the patient's perspective', Carman D and Britten N, ***British Journal of General Practice, 45***, 1995, 485–58

11 ***Counselling in HIV infection and AIDS***, Green J and McCreaner A (eds), Blackwell, 1989, 306

12 See ref 2 above, page 40

13 See ref 2 above, page 234

14 'Should insurance companies have access to patients' medical records? Access should be denied', Lavender H, ***British Medical Journal, 313***, 1996, 286

15 See ref 2 above, page 48

16 See ref 2 above, page 86

17 ***AIDS – a moral issue,*** Almond B (ed), Macmillan, 1996

18 'A confidence betrayed', Cassidy J, ***Nursing Times, 90 (12)***, 1994, 16-17

Acknowledgements

We would like to thank Philippa Matthews for her help and advice in putting this chapter together and Paul Thornton for the *Insurance medical reports... in practice* box.

Anne Damerell and Catti Moss

Philip Hannaford

chapter four

screening and well woman/man measures

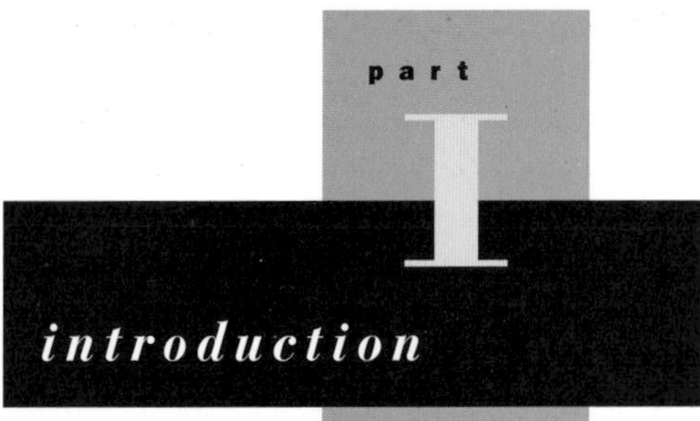

Screening can be defined as the active process of identifying a disease or pre-disease condition in people who are asymptomatic and apparently healthy[1]. Thus, it is very different to the clinical investigation of individuals presenting with symptoms. Most screening procedures do not arise from a person's request for advice for a specific complaint, indeed they are often initiated by the medical profession itself. The ethical considerations of screening, therefore, are different from those applying to traditional curative medicine. A particular concern is the potential to change someone, at least temporarily, from being a supposedly healthy individual to one with disease or potential disease.

This said, perceived wisdom that prevention is better than cure has led to a variety of screening procedures being undertaken in sexual health, family planning and well-person clinics conducted in general practice:

- screening for asymptomatic disease, or markers of risk, in order to maximise the safe provision of treatment, eg screening for sexually transmitted infections (STIs) before inserting an intrauterine device or performing an induced abortion, or for raised blood pressure before prescribing combined oral contraceptives (COCs)
- opportunistic, population or high risk group screening for asymptomatic disease not directly connected with the safe provision of treatment but related to sexual health, eg screening for STIs in adolescents, or cervical cancer screening
- opportunistic, population or high risk group screening for markers of increased risk of disease unrelated to sexual health, eg measuring the blood pressure of all clinic attenders, or screening for cholesterol screening in individuals with a close family history of cardiovascular disease
- opportunistic screening for the absence of protection against disease, eg screening for rubella antibodies in young women, or for hepatitis antibodies in homosexuals and prostitutes

The purpose of the various activities can be different. Sometimes, they are undertaken to avoid causing harm by proposed treatments. In other cases, they are to improve the population's health by using the opportunity of the consultation to provide preventive services to a hopefully receptive group of consumers. A third reason may be a desire to provide reassurance. Determining the underlying purpose for a screening procedure is important. Screening procedures directly related to the provision of safe medical care should take precedence over all others. This differentiation is helpful when deciding how to prioritise the use of scarce resources, and when determining which procedures to leave out if an individual wishes to have the minimum of interventions.

Principles of screening procedures

A classic summary of the requirements of a screening programme appeared in 1968[2], and have not changed materially since[1]. The principles are:

- the condition sought should be an important health problem, usually because it is common and serious
- there should be an accepted treatment for patients with the recognised disease
- facilities for diagnosis and treatment should be available

- there should be a recognisable latent or early symptomatic stage
- there should be a suitable test or examination
- the test should be acceptable to the population
- the natural history of the disease should be adequately understood, and there should be evidence that early diagnosis offers a better outcome than a later one
- there should be an agreed policy about whom to treat as patients
- the cost of case-finding (including diagnosis and treatment of individuals with disease) should be economically balanced in relation to possible expenditure on medical care as a whole
- case-finding should be a continuing process and not a 'once for all' project

Characteristics of a screening test

A *sensitive* screening procedure gives a positive result when the person being screened has the disease of interest; low sensitivity means that the number of false negatives (missed cases) is high. A *specific* screening procedure gives a negative result when the person being screened does not have the disease of interest; low specificity means that the number of false positives (non-cases) is high. The *positive predictive* value of the screening procedure is the proportion of persons with a positive result who actually have the disease. Conversely, the *negative predictive value* is the proportion of individuals with a negative result who do not have the disease. Predictive values of a test are useful as they reflect the underlying prevalence of disease in the community being screened; procedures developed and evaluated in hospital settings usually have very different predictive values when used in the community where the prevalence of disease tends to be lower. A low positive predictive value means that a large number of individuals have to be assessed in order to detect one case.

Costs of screening

The costs of screening can be substantial. Direct costs include the time needed to perform the test or examination, costs of consumable items and laboratory facilities, expenditure investigating individuals with a positive result (who may not necessarily have the disease), and the cost of treating patients finally deemed to have the disease.

Indirect costs are more difficult to quantify but are no less important[3]. Screening can create a false sense of security if a false negative result is obtained. The long interval between exposure and development of a positive test for human immunodeficiency virus (HIV) does not mean that a person with a negative result is clear of the infection. On the other hand, a false positive result can cause increased anxiety which does not necessarily resolve immediately an individual is found to be free of disease. A healthy consumer of preventative services can be turned into a worried patient. In family planning, inappropriate screening may restrict the range of contraceptives available. Not only does this limit choice; it could result in more ill-health. For example, women who are denied COCs because of dubious screening activities will not be able to use a highly effective contraceptive. Nor will they benefit from non-contraceptive advantages of oral contraceptives, including substantial, sustained protection against endometrial and ovarian cancer. Even worse, the need to undergo costly, frightening or embarrassing procedures before receiving contraceptive services may result in some sexually active women not using any method of birth control.

Finally, everything has its opportunity costs; money or time spent on one thing cannot be spent on another. Given the huge numbers of individuals using sexual health-related services, any routine screening procedure will place a heavy burden on health service resources. In family planning clinics, inappropriate screening may leave insufficient time to explain how to use the contraceptive properly or to discuss other aspects of sexual health.

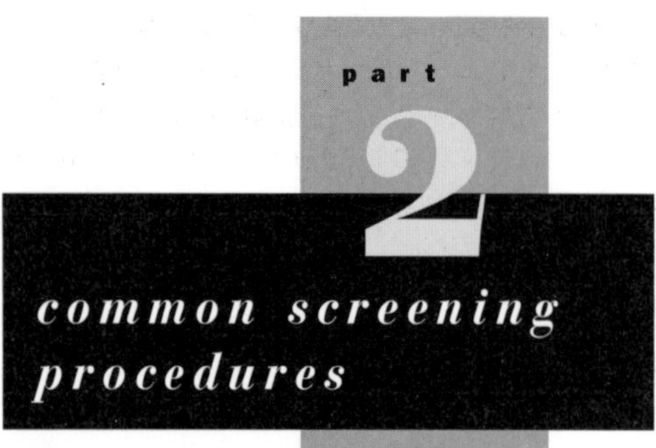

part 2 common screening procedures

This section examines the value of a number of screening procedures commonly performed on people under 50. It is worth noting that the conclusions reached may be different if an older population were being assessed. This is because the sensitivity and specificity of a screening procedure, and the incidence and prevalence of disease, often change with age, thereby altering the value of the test at different ages.

Blood pressure measurement

Research shows strong increasing trends between both diastolic and systolic blood pressure and the risk of coronary heart disease and stroke[4]; and good evidence that effective management substantially reduces this risk[5]. Studies of the effects of COCs continue to show blood pressure increases in some users, even with modern low dose preparations[6]. Furthermore, epidemiological studies have found an enhanced risk of stroke[7,8] and acute myocardial infarction[9,10,11] in users of COCs with a history of hypertension. Although the absolute risk is very small because cardiovascular disease is uncommon in young women, each of these observations indicates a need to measure the blood pressure of women before and during COC use. The widespread availability, and cheapness of the procedure, provide further support for this action.

The most appropriate frequency of monitoring has not been the subject of close scientific scrutiny. An arbitrary recommendation would be that the blood pressure is checked before using COCs, at 1-3 months after starting, then at 6 monthly intervals with perhaps an extension of the interval to annual checks if the blood pressure remains low after two or three years of use[12]. The need to continue blood pressure monitoring is indicated by evidence that some COC users develop increases in blood pressure even after prolonged periods of use[13].

Many clinicians also have a low threshold for measuring the blood pressure of individuals attending for other methods of contraception, or for other reasons. In such circumstances, the clinician is screening for a risk marker of a disease unrelated to sexual health. Opportunistic screening amongst older people is recommended, given the widespread incidence of cardiovascular disease in this age group in the western world, good evidence that effective management substantially reduces the risk, and the availability of a cheap and acceptable screening procedure. Some workplace screening programmes, however, have observed that people found to be hypertensive have increased sick leave, increased anxiety and reduced self-perceived health status, regardless of whether their hypertension warranted treatment[3]. Bearing this in mind, some clinicians may prefer to restrict opportunistic screening below the age of about 40 years to people at high risk of cardiovascular disease: diabetics, smokers, the obese, those with a close family history or with a known lipid abnormality.

Urinalysis

Urinalysis for glucose, blood or protein is not recommended. In young individuals, urine testing for glucose results detects very few undiagnosed diabetics (less than 1 in 1,000); the false positive rate is between 1 and 2 per cent[14]. This low pick-up rate is related to the very low prevalence of asymptomatic disease; screening using blood samples is equally unproductive[14]. As a consequence, the costs per identified case are relatively high[14]. There is no evidence that the early detection and treatment of asymptomatic diabetes improves long-term outcome[15]. Furthermore, since women with uncomplicated diabetes can safely use all methods of contraception, including COCs, the detection of hidden diabetes will not alter patient management.

Similar problems of very low detection rates, relatively high costs, no evidence of long-term benefits from early detection and no contribution to clinical management, affect urinalysis for renal disease[14].

Cervical smears and bimanual pelvic examination

Comprehensive, regular screening for cervical cancer with Papanicalou smears reduces mortality from this disease[16]. Current policy in the UK is for women aged 20 to 64 years to be screened at least every five years[1]. Even with contractual changes which provide incentives for GPs to meet performance targets, there is a small but important proportion of women who have never had a smear. On the other hand, there are many women who have had many more than the recommended number of smears even though they are at low risk of cervical cancer. The important public health benefits of reducing the incidence of, and mortality from, cervical cancer will be achieved more cost-effectively by decreasing the number of inappropriate smears and increasing the participation of women who have never had one. The primary care team has an important, although not unique, role in meeting this challenge.

Studies from several countries show that the highest frequency of pre-invasive conditions (dysplasia or carcinoma-in-situ, collectively called cervical intraepithelial neoplasia (CIN)) occur at 25-35 years of age, with invasive cancer most frequent around 45-50 years[17]. Given the very low proportion of teenage women with pre-invasive lesions, there is no justification for starting routine screening before the age of 20. Current evidence indicates that a three year interval between screening, provides 90 per cent protection against invasive cancer, provided that the test has reasonable sensitivity[17]. A five year screening programme offers approximately 84 per cent protection. Many practices have adopted the shorter, three year interval. When doing so, it is important to recognise that at each stage of progression, perhaps only 15 per cent of lesions transform to a more serious one, while the other 85 per cent either heal spontaneously or remain unchanged[17]. Since we are currently unable to identify which lesions will progress, there is inevitably over-treatment of the condition; excessive screening exacerbates this problem.

Many studies have suggested an important association between use of COCs and an increased risk of dysplasia, carcinoma-in-situ, squamous cell and adeno-carcinoma of the cervix[18]. The association, however, may be due to related factors such as differences in lifestyle and sexual history of women using different methods of birth control, rather than a biological effect of oral contraceptives. There is no strong evidence that hormonal contraceptives of any type accelerate the progress of pre-invasive cervical tumours. Thus, while all users of hormonal contraceptives should participate in the national screening programme, there is no reason for them to be screened more frequently than other women. Similar lack of evidence of acceleration of progress from early pre-invasive stages in women with other risk factors, such as a history of genital warts, means that these women do not need to be screened more frequently than individuals at lower risk[17].

A bimanual pelvic examination is often performed when taking a cervical smear, although the purpose for this procedure is frequently unclear. Bimanual pelvic examinations are not pre-requisite components of a cervical cancer screening programme. If the purpose is to detect ovarian cancer, then the procedure is a poor screening test for it has low sensitivity, cannot distinguish between malignant and benign ovarian cysts, there is no evidence that benign cysts have malignant potential, and the false positive rate is high resulting in low sensitivity[19]. The false positive rate is high even when performed by a gynaecologist, and may be higher still when undertaken by GPs or practice nurses. It is unlikely that the procedure is better at screening for other conditions. The available evidence, therefore, argues strongly against using the bimanual pelvic examination as a routine screening procedure in asymptomatic women.

Screening for breast cancer

So far, eleven studies have examined the value of mammography in women aged less than 50 years; none have demonstrated a statistically significant reduction in mortality[20]. It should be noted, however, that none of the studies were large enough to detect a valuable reduction in mortality. For this reason, two major clinical trials are underway in Europe. Until these trials report, there are no scientific grounds for the routine screening of women aged under 50 by mammography.

Intuitively, breast self-examination is an attractive alternative screening procedure. There is not, however, strong evidence that regular breast self-examination reduces mortality[21]. Most cancers occurring in women who practice the technique are not found during the self examination. Furthermore, the false positive rate is high resulting in many women having unnecessary biopsies. This is especially so in younger women[22]. Breast self-examination is time-consuming to teach properly. For these reasons, the teaching of breast self-examination cannot be recommended. Instead all women should be advised to practice 'breast awareness'. This is part of normal self-care whereby women are alert to any unusual changes in their breasts detected during normal daily activities such as washing and report these changes promptly to the appropriate medical services.

Blood tests in oral contraceptive users

All currently available COCs produce a variety of alterations in carbohydrate, lipid and lipoprotein metabolism, as well as haemostatic changes[23]. The clinical significance of these changes is still unknown. At present, any screening should be restricted to women with a strong personal or family history of venous or arterial vascular disease. (Arbitary definitions of this are: a close relative with venous thromboembolism (VTE) before age 50; with arterial disease before age 65.) In particular the routine testing of all new users for clotting abnormalities is not justified. This is partly because more than 50 per cent of cases cannot be predicted by the currently available assays[24]. The low incidence of VTE complications also means that the predictive value of the tests is low, dramatically increasing the costs of any screening programme. In addition, only a tiny proportion of women with such defects will develop a problem. Since we cannot currently identify which women are at particular risk, and given that there is no specific treatment, the only way to minimise the risk would be to deny COCs to all women with such abnormalities – perhaps 6 per cent of the general population[24].

Cholesterol measurement

Cholesterol measurement is often done to screen for markers of risk of disease unrelated directly to sexual health. There is still no consensus about the value of population screening for raised cholesterol levels. Many clinicians prefer to target the measurement of cholesterol in individuals already at known increased risk of cardiovascular disease rather than undertake the blanket screening of everyone. Tables have been developed for identifying, on the basis of age, smoking habits, history of hypertension and diabetes, and evidence of left ventricular hypertrophy, those in whom the measurement of cholesterol is warranted[25]. The important concept underling these tables, and other devices for determining risk of cardiovascular disease, is the need to consider together all known risk factors rather than act on any one in isolation.

Screening for prostate cancer

Although prostate cancer is the third most common cause of cancer death in men, few cases appear before the age of 50. This said, there is growing interest in screening tests to detect this disease. So far, three methods have been used, sometimes in combination: digital rectal examination, trans-urethral ultrasound and measurements of serum prostate specific antigen (PSA) levels[26]. None has been evaluated in long-term studies to assess its value in reducing mortality from this disease. Raised PSA levels appear to be the more sensitive screening procedure, but only a quarter to one third of asymptomatic men with abnormally high levels are subsequently found to have prostate cancer. The investigations required to confirm the diagnosis of cancer can have important physical and psychological complications, including effects in individuals subsequently not found to have the disease. Furthermore, neither PSA levels nor follow-up biopsies, predict which cancers will progress to cause illness or death. Many of the detected cancers appear to be extremely slow growing, with no impact on the man's health. It is likely, therefore, that many of the detected cancers are overtreated with the potential for adverse physical and psychological effects. Until more is known about the balance of risks and benefits, screening for prostate cancer cannot be recommended[26].

Screening for testicular cancer

In young men, testicular cancer is more common than cancer of the prostate. There is no recognised screening procedure for testicular cancer. Men are instead advised to practice 'testicular awareness' whereby they be alert to any new genital changes and report these promptly to the appropriate medical services for further evaluation.

Rubella antibodies

Maternal rubella infection in the first eight to ten weeks of pregnancy results in fetal damage in up to 90 per cent of infants, with multiple defects common (the Congenital Rubella Syndrome)[27]. Although the number of confirmed cases of Congenital Rubella Syndrome has fallen in recent years, the impact of the condition warrants screening women of child-bearing age for rubella antibodies and immunising those found to be seronegative. Since women attending for family planning services are presumably not wanting to get pregnant in the immediate future, these consultations provide a useful opportunity to screen for rubella antibodies. This approach would avoid immunising a pregnant woman, although there is no evidence that inadvertent immunisation shortly before or during pregnancy is associated with Congenital Rubella Syndrome[27].

To avoid the risk of transmitting rubella to pregnant women, all health service staff (male and female) should be screened and immunised if seronegative.

Hepatitis B antibodies

Hepatitis B is a potentially serious disease with perhaps two to ten per cent of those infected as adults becoming carriers of the virus for more than six months[27]. Chronic carriage is more frequent in those infected as children and rise to 90 per cent in those infected perinatally.

Immunisation is currently recommended for:

- babies born to mothers who are chronic carriers of hepatitis B virus or to mothers who have had acute hepatitis B during pregnancy.
- parental drug misusers
- individuals who change sexual partners frequently, especially gay or bisexual men, and men or women who are prostitutes
- close family contacts of a case or carrier
- families adopting children from countries with a high prevalence of hepatitis B
- haemophiliacs, others regularly receiving blood transfusions or other products, and those carers responsible for administering these products
- patients with chronic renal failure
- health care workers, including students and trainees
- staff and residents of residential accommodation for those with severe learning disabilities (mental handicap)
- some other occupational groups, eg morticians, embalmers, prison staff
- inmates of custodial institutions
- those travelling to areas of high prevalence seeking work or likely to stay there for long periods

In most cases, it is recommended that the immunisation be performed without screening beforehand. The vaccine, however, should not be given to individuals who are already hepatitis B surface antigen positive (because it is unnecessary) or those with acute hepatitis B (because it is ineffective). In some cases, therefore, screening for hepatitis B surface antibodies should be undertaken before offering immunisation. Such groups may include parental drug misusers and individuals who change their sexual partners frequently. Antenatal screening is also recommended for pregnant women in order to identify babies who require immunisation after birth. Limited screening of pregnant women at higher risk of hepatitis B does not identify all disease carriers. Thus, hepatitis B screening should be offered to all women attending antenatal clinics.

Screening for HIV

HIV testing is sought for a variety of reasons:

- to know that the infection has/has not been caught
- to take special care of health (including possibly drug treatment) if HIV is detected
- to inform decisions about whether condom use needs to continue within a stable relationship
- to inform decisions about having children
- because of employment or insurance considerations
- because certain countries requiring testing before entry[28]

In each situation, the person needs to consider:

- exactly why the test is being requested (eg is s/he being put under undue pressure to have one, is there really an increased risk of contracting the infection?)
- how will s/he handle the result (whether negative or positive)
- how will the test result affect any existing/future relationships

The timing of the test is important. Most HIV tests detect antibodies to the virus. The interval between being infected with the virus and developing enough antibodies to register a positive test can be up to three months. Thus, a gap of at least three months needs to be left between exposure and most HIV testing. During this period of sero-conversion, however, the individual still has sufficient virus to infect another person, highlighting the need to continue practising safer sex. Anyone requesting an HIV test requires careful discussion about these, and other issues, beforehand. For many individuals, HIV testing may be best performed in the genitourinary medicine clinic (GUM or STI clinic) or, if available, local specialist HIV clinics.

Screening for STIs

Pelvic infection, infertility, ectopic pregnancy and chronic pelvic pain are important long-term sequelae of STIs. Some infections, such as Chlamydia trachomatis, are often asymptomatic, increasing the chance of spread and subsequent tubal damage.

Practices wishing to undertake screening for STIs need to be aware of:

- client factors likely to indicate greater risk of infection
- the prevalence of infection in their population (ideally)
- the strengths and limitations of the locally recommended screening tests
- any practical issues about taking, storing and transporting the specimen
- how to notify clients of the results and deal with any of the difficult and sensitive issues which can arise
- how to provide an efficient tracing service for partners of clients with positive results
- the current local recommendations for treatment.

Close liaison with the local microbiological laboratory and the GUM department is strongly recommended.

Selective screening based on reported risk factors is likely to be the most cost-effective approach to screening general practice attenders.

At present, there is uncertainty about the precise role of screening for STIs in asymptomatic people attending for sexual health services. The Royal College of Obstetricians and Gynaecologists recently recommended, as an alternative to prophylactic antibiotics, screening for chlamydia, gonorrhoea and bacterial vaginosis prior to an induced abortion, or before other uterine instrumentation in non-pregnant women aged less than 35 years (eg IUD insertion, infertility laparoscopy, endometrial sampling)[29]. Only a policy of screening offers the possibility of tracing and treating partners of infected women, thereby reducing the chances of re-infection. Interest in screening for chlamydia exists because the sequelae of the infection are more serious for women than men and studies have consistently reported high prevalence rates in asymptomatic, sexually active women aged under 25. A multidisciplinery expert advisory group on Chlamydia trachomatis has been convened by the Chief Medical Officer to provide further guidance on who should be screened for chlamydia and in which settings. Its report should provide further guidance on the role of screening for chlamydia in primary care.

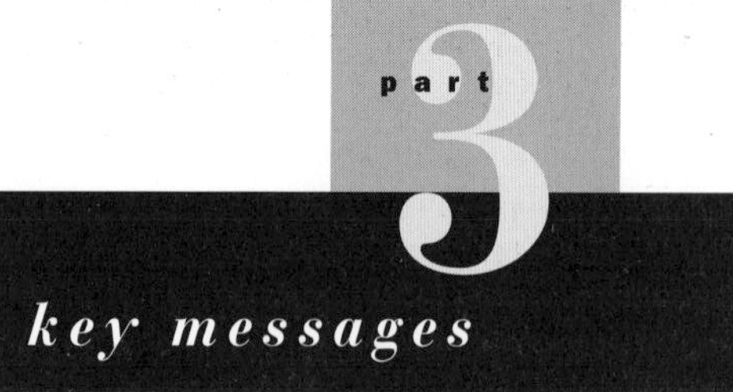

- **Screening offers the potential both to produce benefits and cause harm**
- **Providers of sexual health services need to be clear about the purpose of each screening procedure, its benefits and disadvantages, who should be offered the test and what to do if the results are negative, positive or equivocal**

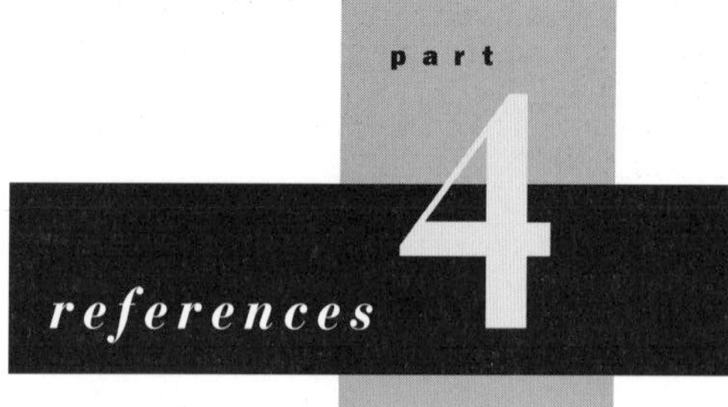

1 ***Screening in health care***, Holland WW and Stewart S, Nuffield Provincial Hospitals Trust, 1990

2 ***Principles and practice of screening for disease***, Wilson JMG and Junger G, World Health Organization, Geneva, 1968

3 'Screening could seriously damage your health', Stewart-Brown S and Farmer A, ***British Medical Journal, 314***, 1997, 533-34

4 'Blood pressure, stroke and coronary heart disease: Part 1, prolonged differences in blood pressure: prospective observational studies corrected for regression dilution bias', MacMahon S, Peto R and Cutler J, et al, ***The Lancet, 335,*** 1990, 765-74

5 'Blood pressure, stroke and coronary heart disease: Part 2, short-term reductions in blood pressure: overview of randomised drug trials in their epidemiological context', Collins R, Peto R and MacMahon, et al, ***The Lancet, 335,*** 1990, 827-38

6 'Effect of four combined oral contraceptives on blood pressure in the pill-free interval', Nichols M, Robinson G and Bounds W, et al, ***Contraception, 47,*** 1993, 367-76

7 'Oral contraceptives and stroke in young women, Collaborative Group for the Study of Stroke in Young Women', ***Journal of the American Medical Association, 231,*** 1975, 718-22

8 'Haemorrhagic stroke, overall stroke risk, and combined oral contraceptives: results of an international, multi-centre, case-control study', WHO Collaborative Study of Cardiovascular Disease and Steroid Hormone Contraception, ***The Lancet, 348,*** 1996, 505-10

9 'Medical progress: oral contraceptives and cardiovascular disease', Stadel BV, ***New England Journal of Medicine, 305,*** 1981, 672-77

10 'Risk factors for acute myocardial infarction in women: evidence from the Royal College of General Practitioners' Oral Contraception Study, Croft P and Hannaford PC, ***British Medical Journal, 298,*** 1989, 165-68

11 'Acute myocardial infarction and combined oral contraceptives: results from an international multicentre case-control study', WHO Collaborative Study of Cardiovascular Disease and Steroid Hormone Contraception, ***The Lancet, 349,*** 1997, 1202-09

12 ***Evidence-guided prescribing of the pill***, Hannaford PC and Webb AMC (eds), 'Oral contraceptives and blood pressure', Poulter NR, Parthenon Publishing Group 1996, 77-88

13 'Blood pressure in women taking oral contraceptives', Weir RJ, Briggs E, and Mack A, et al, ***British Medical Journal, 1,*** 1974, 533-35

14 ***Evidence-guided prescribing of the pill***, Hannaford PC and Webb AMC (eds), 'The appropriateness of urinalysis as a routine screening test before oral contraceptive prescription', Thorogood M and Langham S, Parthenon Publishing Group 1996, 251-62

15 'Urine analysis for glucose and protein: are the requirements of the new contract sensible?', Mant D and Fowler G, ***British Medical Journal, 300***, 1990, 1053-55

16 'Cancer: causes, occurrence and control', ***IARC Scientific Publication No 100***, Tomatis L (ed), WHO International Agency for Research on Cancer, 1990

17 ***Evidence-guided prescribing of the pill***, Hannaford PC and Webb AMC (eds), 'Cervical smears: when to start and how often to do', Buiatti E, Parthenon Publishing Group, 1996, 157-66

18 ***Evidence-guided prescribing of the pill***, Hannaford PC and Webb AMC (eds), 'The association between oral contraceptive use and neoplasia of the cervix, vagina and vulva', Irwin KL, Parthenon Publishing Group, 1996, 145-56

19 ***Evidence-guided prescribing of the pill***, Hannaford PC and Webb AMC (eds), 'Screening for ovarian cancer', Austoker J, Parthenon Publishing Group 1996, 167-73

20 ***Evidence-guided prescribing of the pill***, Hannaford PC and Webb AMC (eds), 'Screening for breast cancer in young women', Cuckle H, Parthenon Publishing Group, 1996, 209-15

21 ***Evidence-guided prescribing of the pill***, Hannaford PC and Webb AMC (eds), 'Screening for breast cancer in young women using breast self-examination', Hackshaw AK, Parthenon Publishing Group, 1996, 217-26

22 'Breast self examination: should we discourage it?', Mant D, ***British Journal of General Practice, 39,*** 1989, 180-81

23 'Consensus development meeting 1995: combined oral contraceptives and cardiovascular disease', The Writing Committee for the Second European Conference on Sex Steroids and Metabolism, ***Gynecological Endocrinology, 10,*** 1996, 1-5

24 ***Evidence-guided prescribing of the pill,*** Hannaford PC and Webb AMC (eds), 'Role of screening for vascular disease in pill users: the haemostatic system', Winkler UH, Parthenon Publishing Group 1996, 109-20

25 'The Sheffield table for primary prevention of coronary heart disease: corrected', Ramsay LE, Haq IU and Jackson PR, et al, ***The Lancet, 348,*** 1996, 1251-52

26 'Screening for prostate cancer', ***Effectiveness Matters, 1997,*** vol 2, issue 2, NHS Centre for Reviews and Dissemination

27 ***Immunisation against infectious diseases,*** Salisbury DM and Begg NT (eds), HMSO, 1996

28 ***Testing issues: a booklet for people thinking of having an HIV test,*** Terrence Higgins Trust, 1996

29 ***Recommendations arising from the 31st study group: the prevention of pelvic infection,*** Templeton A (ed), RCOG Press, 1996

Trefor Lloyd

Joan Walsh

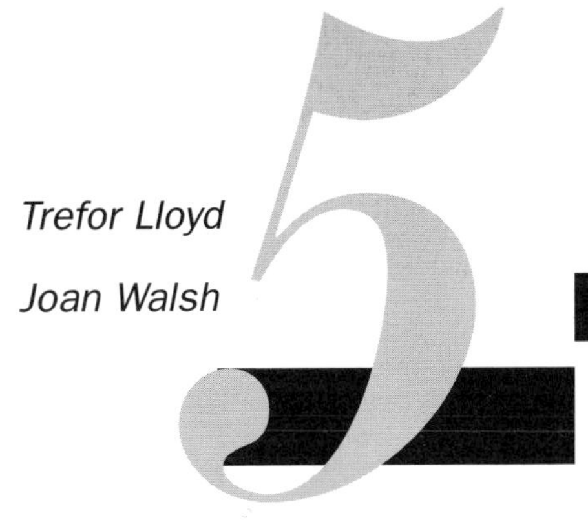

chapter five

men's issues in sexual health

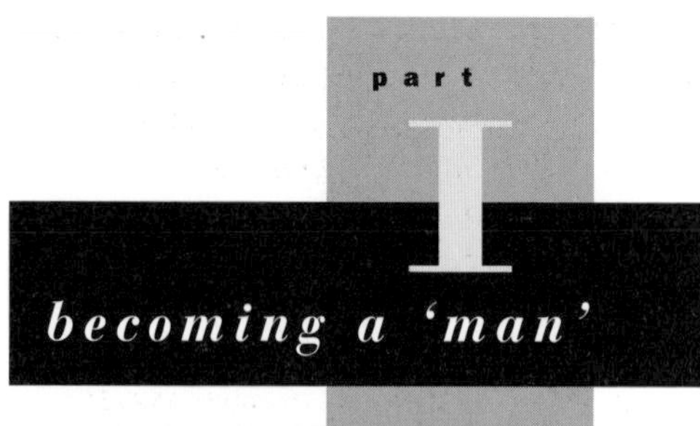

'... becoming a man is a complex process of learning and doing within shifting sets of social constraints'[1]

Whether they identify as gay, bisexual or heterosexual, most men will have been socialised to be 'male'. Unfortunately, in this culture, male gender socialisation can have the effect of reducing both men's ability to maintain and protect their own health (including sexual health) and their willingness to use health services.

In his 1992 report, the Chief Medical Officer[2] noted that men and women consistently show different patterns of mortality, morbidity and health service use, and that there is

'increasing evidence that many of the patterns observed stem from differences in health-related behaviour, which may be influenced by the knowledge, attitudes and beliefs of men. For example, men seem to be less aware of the impact of certain behaviours on their health'.

The CMO's report further observes that

'studies of health related behaviour indicate that considerable gains may be achieved by specific targeting of messages to improve men's general knowledge about health and more specifically to improve their awareness of the links between their own behaviour and its health consequences. Unfortunately the same attitudes and behaviours that put men at greater risk also tend to make them less accessible to health promotion messages'

These 'attitudes and behaviours' reflect the way that men learn what it is to be masculine. For example, boys and young men learn to:

- appear to be 'strong' by keeping feelings and emotions inside
- avoid showing any signs of physical or emotional 'weakness' or vulnerability
- protect themselves by being in control and appearing 'cool' – emotionally detached and uninvolved
- at all costs avoid being ridiculed by peers and 'losing face'
- disregard health and health needs
- continue to prove their masculinity by conforming to heterosexual 'macho' cultures and values – eg responding aggressively to provocation, being sexist, being homophobic, taking active and passive risks[3-5]

Given this social context, it is not surprising that men use health care services only *in extremis,* rather than in a precautionary or preventative way – approaching a health care professional is likely to involve a course of action which is particularly difficult for men because it directly contradicts notions of masculinity, for example:

- admitting to another person that you may have a problem, and one that you can't solve yourself
- asking for help
- admitting that you are worried/anxious about your health (or about someone else's)
- talking about yourself, your signs and symptoms, your fears and concerns, your feelings
- admitting that there are things that you don't know or know about
- having beliefs, attitudes and behaviours, including risk-taking, questioned/challenged
- giving up power and control of the situation

For all the reasons outlined above (and no doubt many others) men can be 'hard to reach' – *but men's low uptake of primary health care services can never be assumed to mean a 'lack of demand'.*

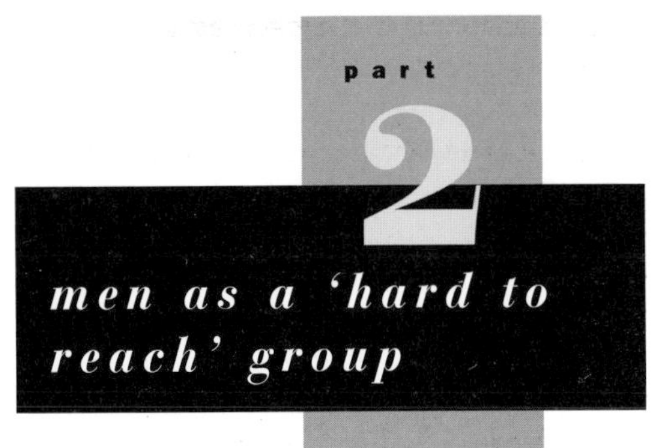

part 2 men as a 'hard to reach' group

In a research project in 1994 which audited provision of sexual health services for heterosexual men, Davidson and Lloyd[6] found a number of possible reasons for poor uptake:

- heterosexual men resist using HIV/AIDS services because they still see these as being for gay men, ie their homophobia inhibits them from using services that are open to all
- when men do use services, it is because they do so as part of some other aspect of their identity, eg as black men, as men with a disability, or survivors of abuse. They do not tend to use services that are 'for men'
- many services are daytime only, and working men have difficulty in taking time off work to use them. To do so would make them visible to others as having a 'problem'; and, importantly
- the 'disease focus' of many services puts many men off

Services which do appear to be used by heterosexual men include:

- services which allow self-referral, and which allow men to retain 'control'
- services offered by groups of highly motivated men (eg self-help voluntary groups) committed to helping others in similar situations
- crisis intervention/management services
- workplace-based services, eg workplace 'well man' screening services
- telephone helplines which offer anonymity
- campaigns which target places where men gather (eg pubs, clubs, sports grounds)
- those which put the emphasis on 'fitness' and 'health', not 'illness' or 'disease'

Men seem to respond to a concrete, practical service which has a clearly defined and accurately described purpose, so that they know what they can expect before approaching – eg 'free condoms'. But services should always be prepared to meet other needs – whatever is specifically on the health promotion agenda, work with men is likely to lead to discussion of wider sexual health and emotional/relationship issues. Men may also be willing to address relationship difficulties and the broader aspects of sexual health in another guise, by another name – for example, 'assertiveness' or 'stress management'.

Increasing uptake of sexual health services for men means:

- recognising the barriers to sexual health created by the male gender role
- recognising that men's socialisation will affect their response to any form of intervention – what looks like machismo is just as likely to be embarrassment
- creating opportunities for all men to identify and discuss their sexual health needs
- adopting a positive and practical approach to sexual health service provision for men
- working to ensure that service environment and staff team attitudes are 'male-friendly'
- targeting and marketing information and services for men effectively

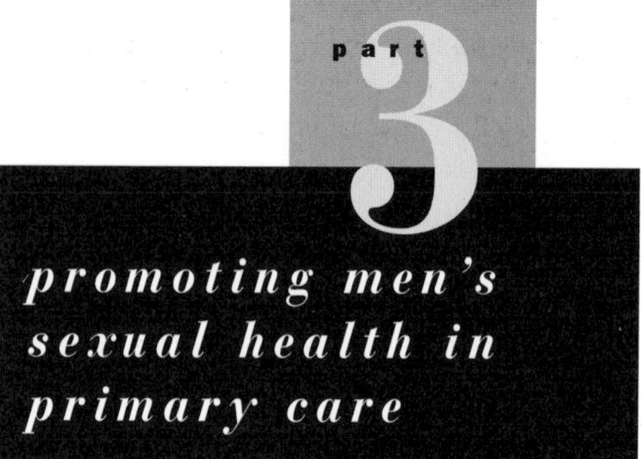

part 3 promoting men's sexual health in primary care

Because men tend not to use primary health care consultations in a precautionary or preventative way, opportunities for opportunistic health promotion may appear limited. Undertaking sexual health promotion may be further constrained by the need to ask men to discuss intensely personal and perhaps taboo subjects like sex, sexuality, sexual behaviour, sexual experiences and relationships.

In some consultations, for example when a man attends with symptoms of sexually transmitted disease, discussion of these issues may be more obviously legitimate and so easier. This may also be a time when men are more than usually receptive to health information and advice. On the other hand, when men do attend in such circumstances, they may want only to deal with the presenting problem and (ideally) to be offered a 'quick fix' rather than discussing behavioural change. This 'agenda' may be reinforced by professional expectations of men and of consultations with men.

Working successfully with men to promote sexual health means:

- being prepared to take the initiative, expecting to take the time and planning the follow up
- being consistent and being persistent
- working with the 'positive and responsible' (he has overcome the barriers and approached a health professional for help) rather than the 'negative and irresponsible' (he had unprotected sex and has a sexually transmitted infection)
- Promoting sexual health within primary care may also involve recognising the limitations of a reactive service. All available data suggests that primary health care services are not well used by men – the challenge is to find new ways of encouraging men to approach services, and to develop new ways for services to approach men.

For example:

- knowing exactly which boys, young men and adult men you want/need to work with – who are they, what their needs are, what motivates them to use services and what deters them
- creating opportunities for sexual health promotion with men who do already use primary health care services – for example, 'MOTs' with the emphasis on 'health' and 'fitness' and a results format which appeals to men
- taking services to the target group(s) – consider workplace clinics and outreach services in places where men spend time locally, get involved in school sex education programmes to teach boys and young men about their sexual health and about using sexual health services
- making links with other agencies which men use – other statutory and voluntary sector organisations, self-help groups, men's organisations, pressure groups
- targeting information about services directly – target men, not (for example) their partners
- promoting services – being explicit in publicising exactly what services for men are on offer locally, when and where they are, who provides them and who can use them

Of course, within the target group 'men' there will be lots of different sub-groups and it may be necessary to develop local priorities, working strategically and in collaboration with other local sexual and reproductive health services.

In setting out the aims and objectives of any intervention which targets men, bear in mind that the most valuable outcome might be to enable men to acknowledge their health needs and to approach health services for information and advice before the situation reaches crisis point. 'Well man' screening, for example, might not appear to represent 'value for money' or be 'cost effective' if evaluations overlook these wider, and very important, objectives and outcomes.

part 4 *safer sex: men's approaches to condom use and contraception*

Research consistently shows that men's approaches to condom use and contraception tend to be situational and thus inconsistent.

Reasons given by gay and bisexual men for not always using condoms as an element of safer sex include:

- got carried away
- none available
- too drunk (or stoned)
- partner refused
- don't like interruption
- loss of sensitivity
- presumed same HIV status as partner
- only use with casual partners
- uncomfortable

Knowledge may or may not be translated into behaviour, depending on the particular circumstances and context of any encounter – certainly the likelihood of condom use does not depend on knowledge alone. The status of the relationship is an important determinant, as is the level of trust between partners: gay men are more likely always to use condoms with casual partners than with regular partners or within monogamous relationships[7].

Similarly, qualitative research commissioned by the Contraceptive Education Service suggests that the perceived status of the relationship (for example, a 'one-off', casual, ongoing), the degree of perceived risk and the level of trust all influence heterosexual men's attitudes and behaviour with respect to condom use and contraceptive responsibility. In discussion groups condom use was generally reported as being most likely with 'one-off' or otherwise 'risky' partners, and as being abandoned at the earliest opportunity.

Three broadly different approaches to contraceptive responsibility and condom use were described by heterosexually active men – 'passive', 'opportunistic' and 'prepared'. The 'opportunistic' approach was most commonly reported, and is characterised by:

- having some knowledge and being aware of the potential risks and consequences of unprotected sex
- having a sense of personal responsibility for protecting self and partner from unintended paternity/pregnancy and sexually transmitted infection and recognition of the value of using condoms, *but*
- lacking confidence in taking the initiative in raising the issue of contraception and condom use with a partner
- lacking confidence in carrying and using condoms and so adopting an inconsistent approach to contraceptive responsibility
- continuing to take risks with contraception and sexual health, although experiencing anxiety and regret 'the morning after'

In contrast, the 'passive' approach is characterised by feeling remote and removed from the risks and consequences of unprotected sex, little sense of self-preservation and unwillingness to use condoms unless a partner insists or is perceived as particularly 'risky'. At the other extreme, the 'prepared' approach is adopted by men who have a realistic understanding of the consequences of unprotected sex, who always carry and use condoms, and who report feeling entirely confident about discussing contraception and condom use with partners – but an initially strong commitment to shared responsibility for contraception declines as relationships become more established[8].

It is important to note that these are categories of *approach*, not categories of *men*.

Men can and do move between the different approaches, depending on the circumstances of an encounter/relationship and on what else is happening in their lives – which means that there *are* opportunities for health promotion work. Some men will need information about risks, consequences and the value of self-preservation, presented from a male perspective and in a way which is relevant and meaningful. Others may already have the knowledge, but will need support in translating what they know into what they do.

Working successfully with the individual will depend on first establishing 'where he is' – for example, using the above framework, is his current approach to contraception and condom use most likely to be passive, opportunistic or prepared? What, in his mind, are the barriers to consistent condom/contraceptive use? What would motivate him towards a more 'prepared' approach?

The primary care team can work with men to:

- reinforce and build on existing knowledge and understanding
- sustain motivation for adopting consistent approach to contraceptive use in practice – identify practical risk-reduction strategies which don't depend on one-off judgements about people and situations
- focus on practical communication skills and concerns – when and how to talk about using a condom, how to ask whether she is using contraception

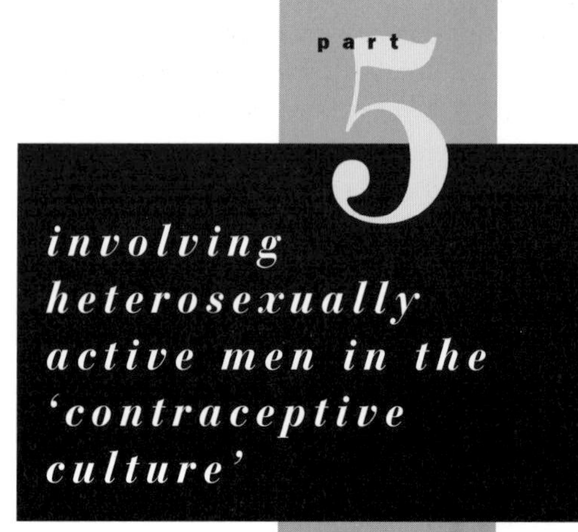

part 5 involving heterosexually active men in the 'contraceptive culture'

There are many arguments for including men in contraceptive provision:

- it is important for men to know how to use male-controlled methods correctly (as a primary and 'back up' method) and to have the confidence to take the initiative in using them
- contraception begins with communication – between men, women and health professionals
- no matter which partner is using a particular contraceptive service/method, both are dependent on that service/method to control their fertility – and both have a right to high quality care
- cultural constraints and professional practices may make it hard for men to ask for information and advice – professionals have a responsibility to ensure that men are not excluded
- men's contraceptive knowledge, attitudes and behaviours can substantially influence women's use of contraception – a well-informed, motivated and confident man is more likely to communicate with his partner and support her use of contraception
- creating opportunities for clients to discuss their experiences of contraceptive methods and services means that the primary health care team can offer practical solutions to any difficulties men may have in using

contraception correctly and consistently. For example, men give 'loss of sensitivity' as a reason for not using condoms, but further discussion may reveal that there is an underlying fear of losing an erection while 'fiddling about'. Onward referral to other staff members (eg for condom teaching) or to other services (eg a health adviser working in genitourinary medicine) may be appropriate

- the 'male pill', or an equivalent, just might become a clinical reality – men may be the family planning clients of the future!

In ensuring that the contraceptive service responds positively to men the primary health care team may need to overcome a number of 'internal barriers' which may reflect public and professional cultures.

For example:

- assumptions and negative stereotypes of men:

'men aren't interested in contraception'
'men don't need to know about contraception'
'there's no point talking to men about contraception – men don't take the pill';
'men won't take responsibility – they don't get pregnant'

- low expectations of men in general, and of their willingness to share responsibility for contraception in particular
- a belief that heterosexual men are a 'lost cause' when it comes to behavioural change

Routinely including men in contraceptive care means taking a positive approach, being willing to take the initiative and helping men make make the most of opportunities to discuss their needs and concerns.

It may be useful to audit existing practice – for example:

- Is contraception routinely discussed with heterosexually active men – for example, when they attend for new patient health checks or other consultations/clinics?
- Does sexual history taking adequately identify men at risk of unintended paternity?
- Does discussion of contraception with men go beyond a recommendation to 'use condoms'?
- When condoms are provided, does provision include information about how to use them, as appropriate, and a demonstration?
- When men attend family planning clinic appointments with a partner, how are they included in the consultation?
- Is the availability of contraceptive information, advice and services actively promoted to men? If so, how?
- What is the uptake of contraceptive information, advice and services by local men?

Professionals may avoid asking men about contraception because, for example, they are anxious about whether they have the necessary skills to work with men, or are concerned about how men will react. But creating opportunities for men to talk about contraception is a vital aspect of sexual health provision and promotion – not least because it challenges, rather than reinforces, the idea that contraception is irrelevant to men. Make it routine to ask all heterosexually active men about contraception – whatever the reaction, you'll get information you can work with.

part 6
key messages

- **Men use primary care services less often and less effectively than women, usually seeking treatment for signs and symptoms. Men rarely use primary care services preventatively**
- **Men's use of health services, the way that men as individuals learn to portray themselves, and cultural beliefs and stereotypes about 'what men are like' combine to make men relatively inaccessible to health professionals**
- **Promoting uptake of primary care services by men is an important dimension of sexual health provision and promotion, having the potential to substantially benefit the health of men and women**
- **Men's approaches to safer sex, condom use and contraception tend to be situational and, consequently, inconsistent. By targeting information and services, and by working positively with men, the primary health care team is ideally placed to motivate men to identify their sexual health and contraceptive needs, and to adopt a more consistent approach to protecting their own and their partners' sexual and reproductive health**

part 7
references

1 ***Wimp or gladiator: contradictions in acquiring masculine sexuality***, Holland J, Ramazanoglu C and Sharpe C, Tufnell Press, 1993

2 ***On the state of the public health***, Calman K, HMSO, 1993, 105

3 ***Recreating sexual politics: men, feminism and politics***, Seidler VJ, Routledge, 1991

4 'Schooling from a masculinities perspective', Seidler VJ, ***What next for men?,*** Lloyd T and Wood T (eds), Working with Men, 1996, 113-26

5 'Why do men want to be victims?', Young K, ***What next for men?,*** Working with Men, 1996, 211-18.

6 ***Working with heterosexual men on sexual health***, Lloyd T and Davidson N, Health Education Authority, 1994

7 ***The sexual lifestyles of gay and bisexual men in England and Wales***, Weatherburn P, Hunt A and Hickson F, et al, Project Sigma, 1992

8 ***It takes two – creating opportunities for clients, Training materials: sexual health, contraception and men,*** Contraceptive Education Service, Health Education Authority, 1997

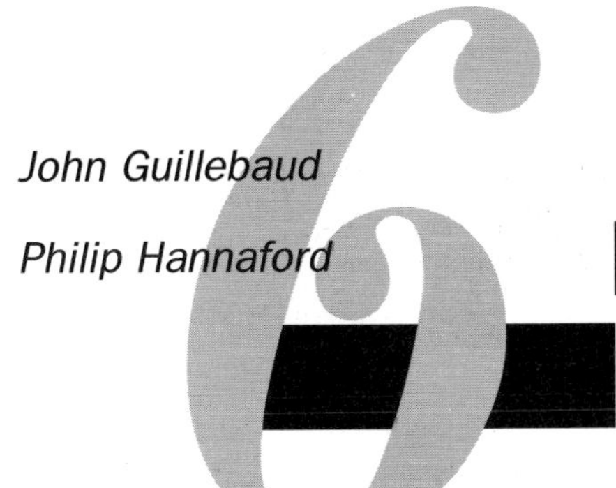

John Guillebaud

Philip Hannaford

chapter six

providing high quality contraceptive services in primary care

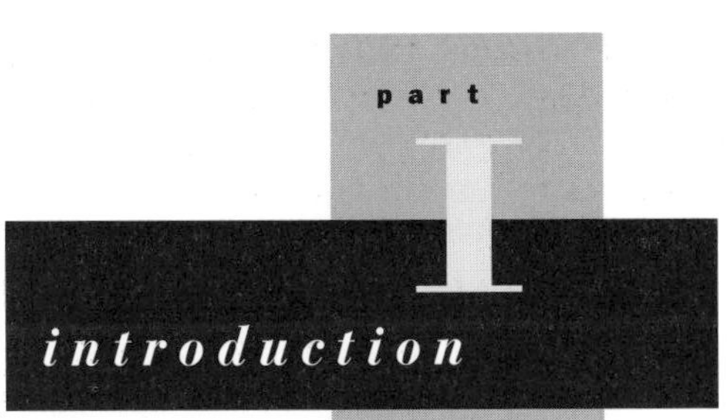

part I introduction

In this chapter we have summarised the main issues that need to be considered when providing contraceptive advice. In recent years several groups of experts have re-examined the evidence on medical criteria for different aspects of contraception[1,2] and we have used this expertise when writing this chapter. In particular, we have made extensive use of a document from the World Health Organization, *Improving access to quality care in family planning: medical eligibility criteria for contraceptive use*[1]. In doing so, we recognise that some of the information may be slightly different to other guidelines published in the UK and elsewhere. The WHO document is explicitly evidence-based.

In this handbook it is assumed that all women can use a method of contraception, unless there are specific reasons to think otherwise. The number of conditions which limit the use of a particular contraceptive is usually small. Using the WHO document, our own experience and advice from other specialists, we have specified:

DO NOT USE WITH THESE CONDITIONS
Conditions which represent an unacceptable health risk if the contraceptive method is used (marked with ● in Table 1, see pages 104–105).

USE CAUTIOUSLY WITH THESE CONDITIONS
Conditions where the theoretical or proven risks usually outweigh the advantages of the method, ie careful clinical judgement is needed, taking into account the severity of the condition and the availability, practicability and acceptability of an alternative method. Usually the method under consideration would be of last choice, and careful follow-up is required. Specialist advice may be needed by the primary care team if a woman has one of these conditions (marked with ◗ in Table 1).

BROADLY USABLE WITH THESE CONDITIONS
Conditions where the advantages of the method generally outweigh any theoretical or proven risks, ie such conditions do not restrict the use of a method but would be a consideration in its selection; careful follow-up may also be needed (marked with ❍ in Table 1).

NB. If a condition is not mentioned then all contraceptive methods can be safely used by affected individuals.

This information is summarised for reversible methods in Table 1 (pages 104–105). For some conditions, caution is only necessary while the problem is being treated (eg avoidance of combined oral contraceptives while a woman has active hepatitis). In other situations, the balance of risks and benefits is different when the condition is known about *before* using a particular contraceptive compared with situations when the condition develops *during* usage. Some cautions are based on theoretical rather than proven risk. Within a particular method, different devices may have different considerations. For these reasons, it is important to consider the more detailed information in the separate sections on each method.

We have not given here our personal preferences about individual or groups of products within each contraceptive method. Consensus is often difficult; in addition, choices change (sometimes very rapidly) in the light of new information. The availability of as comprehensive a range of preparations as possible is important for tailoring choices to the individual needs of each user.

In general, brevity requires us to omit practical details of what to do if problems arise during use of the chosen contraceptive. Much practical advice on these matters exists in the *Contraception today*[3], *FPA contraceptive handbook*[4], *Contraception – your questions answered*[5] and the *Handbook of family planning and reproductive health care*[6].

See Table 1, pages 104–105.

The primary care team has a central role in the provision of contraceptive services in the United Kingdom. The team is often well-placed to offer good advice as it already knows the individual's health and circumstances. While many practices offer excellent services, others provide only indifferent standards of care.

A model of good practice for contraceptive services in primary care includes:

- easy access to services with guaranteed patient confidentiality
- an unhurried consultation with knowledgable personnel, conducted in clean surroundings
- the provision of comprehensive information, tailored to the needs of each individual or couple so that correct choices are made
- the provision of a full range of contraceptive methods (even if this means liaising with outside agencies)
- appropriate assessment before, and monitoring during, use of a particular method in order to minimise any real or perceived adverse effects
- supplementary written information for future reference about the correct use of the chosen method (the UK Family Planning Association Contraceptive Education Service leaflets are particularly recommended)
- information about who to contact if problems or concerns arise about the chosen contraceptive in the future
- consideration of other aspects of sexual health including the need for: protection against sexually transmitted infections (STIs), addressing psychosexual problems, well-person screening
- review of chosen method to check that it remains the most appropriate choice
- full use of the different skills, training and resources of each member of the primary care team – the (well trained) practice nurse perhaps deserving a special mention

The challenge is to enable all service users to feel that they have made the appropriate choice for their circumstances, in an informed and unhurried manner. Sometimes other pressures of everyday general practice – especially time pressures – seem to undermine efforts to meet this challenge. Nonetheless, many practices show on a continuing basis that with good organisation of appropriate human and material resources, it can be done.

The provision of at least one weekly dedicated family planning session assists with dealing with first visits, women with more complex contraceptive problems and those wishing to use methods, such as diaphragms, implants or intrauterine devices and systems (IUDs and IUSs), which initially require more time.

part 3

method of choice

Decisions about the choice of contraception involve a number of considerations: the effectiveness of each method, its perceived safety, recognised contraindications, acceptability, ease of use and availability. Social and cultural influences are also important, as are reversibility issues. The contraceptive options for family spacing are different to those for family limitation (having no more children).

Thus, most contraceptive users are likely to use more than one method during their lifetime. Indeed, for some women such as those not in a stable long-term relationship, active encouragement might need to be given for the simultaneous use of two methods: oral contraceptives to prevent pregnancy and a male or female condom to prevent the spread of STIs. At the end of the day though, choice is dependent on confidence with both the method selected and the service provider (the second of which is related directly to the provision and standard of care).

part 4

relative effectiveness of available methods

The reliability of each method of contraception depends on its inherent effectiveness when used under ideal conditions, and the ability of the couple to use it correctly and consistently in everyday life[7]. 'Iatrogenic' pregnancies are also frequently caused by omissions and errors on the part of service providers – and these are by definition avoidable. Table 2 lists the failure rates quoted in the *FPA contraceptive handbook*[4].

See Tables 2 and 3, page 106

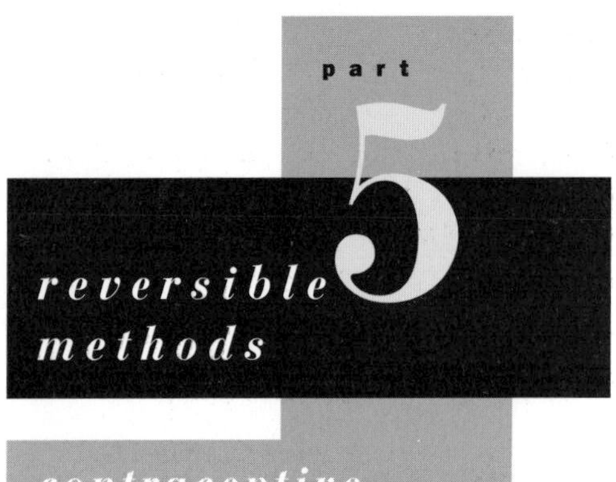

Description

Long-acting progestogens given by deep intramuscular injection; depot medroxyprogesterone acetate (DMPA; Depo-Provera) is given every 12 weeks; norethisterone oenanthate (Noristerat) is licensed to be repeated once only after 8 weeks. Main action: inhibition of ovulation

Advantages

- Highly effective, non-intercourse related contraceptive
- Can often be used by women with conditions which preclude the use of COCs, such as a history of venous thrombosis
- Does not interfere with breast-feeding
- May be particularly advantageous in women with a history of venous thrombosis, endometriosis or sickle cell disease
- Reduced risk of endometrial cancer (DMPA)

Disadvantages

- Once given any side effects are irreversible for the remaining duration of action (ie up to 2-3 months)
- Temporary delay in return of fertility with DMPA (median 9 months after last injection)
- Irregular bleeding, including excessive and more frequent
- Amenorrhoea (DMPA rather than Noristerat)
- Weight gain (DMPA rather than Noristerat)
- Hormonal contraceptives containing progestogen-only have not been widely used, but the pattern of risk of breast cancer with time since last use appears similar to that found for combined oral contraceptives[8].

Do not use with these conditions

- Pregnancy
- Unexplained vaginal bleeding (important to exclude serious underlying illness, especially before initiating use of an injection)
- Current breast cancer

Use cautiously with these conditions

- Breast-feeding less than 6 weeks postpartum (theoretical concern about effects of neonatal exposure to steroids during this period; bleeding irregularities more common)
- Blood pressure 180+/110+mm Hg, or hypertension with vascular disease
- Diabetes *with* nephropathy/retinopathy/neuropathy/other vascular disease, or duration more than 20 years
- Current and history of ischaemic heart disease
- Stroke
- Breast cancer: past history with no evidence of current disease for at least 5 years
- Active viral hepatitis
- Severe (decompensated) liver cirrhosis
- Liver tumours (benign and malignant)

Broadly usable with these conditions

- Before age 16 (theoretical concerns about hypo-oestrogenic effects and interference in future menstrual cycle)
- Questionable fertility from whatever reason
- Blood pressure between 140-180/90-110mm Hg
- Diabetes without vascular disease
- Known hyperlipidaemias
- Abnormal vaginal bleeding patterns: irregular without heavy bleeding, or with heavy or prolonged bleeding (including regular patterns)
- History of combined oral contraceptive (COC)-related cholestasis
- Mild (compensated) liver cirrhosis
- Use of drugs which affect (induce) liver enzymes: rifampicin, rifabutin, griseofulvin, phenytoin, carbamazepine, barbiturates, primidone, topiramate, ritonavir – if used shorten the injection interval to 10 weeks

Initial assessment prior to injection

A careful personal and family medical history with particular attention to cardiovascular risk factors, and an accurate blood pressure measurement is sufficient for most women. Further assessment is needed only if a relevant personal or family history is disclosed, or the blood pressure is very severely elevated. Future pregnancy intentions should also be asked about, especially whether the user wishes to get pregnant immediately after the injection becomes ineffective (DMPA is associated with a temporary delay in return to fertility). There is no need for routine screening by means of physical examination (including breast and bimanual pelvic examination), urine or blood test, before using a contraceptive injection. Indeed, the routine use of such procedures can restrict accessibility to use of an injection, as well as other methods of contraception.

Monitoring during usage

The follow-up assessment should include enquiries about any problems, especially the development of new or more severe headaches and an assessment of any abnormal bleeding patterns. Many practitioners check blood pressure before every injection although there is little evidence on which to base this practice. Little is known about the effects of contraceptive injections on a user's blood pressure. If the next injection is more than 7 days overdue, then the contraceptive benefits are lost.

contraceptive implants

Description

Six polydimethylsiloxane implants, each releasing small amounts of levonorgestrel (Norplant); effect lasting for 5 years

Main effects: inhibition of ovulation (especially during first 3 years of use), changes in cervical mucus making it hostile to sperm penetration, endometrial changes

Advantages

- Highly effective, non-intercourse related contraceptive
- Can often be used by women with conditions which preclude the use of COCs, such as a history of venous thrombosis
- Biological effects less than progestogen-only injections; more like progestogen-only pill (POP)
- Does not interfere with breast-feeding

Disadvantages

- Once given any side effects are irreversible until rods are removed
- Irregular bleeding, including excessive, prolonged, more frequent, especially in first few months
- Insertion requires small surgical procedure under local anaesthetic; *potential* risk of infection, migration of rods, difficulties with removal
- Reported side effects include acne, nausea, headaches, hair loss and hair growth

Do not use with these conditions

- Pregnancy
- Unexplained vaginal bleeding (important to exclude serious underlying illness, especially before inserting Norplant)
- Current breast cancer
- Allergy to levonorgestrel

Use cautiously with these conditions

- Breast-feeding less than 6 weeks postpartum (theoretical concern about effects of neonatal exposure to steroids during this period; bleeding irregularities more common)
- Current and history of ischaemic heart disease, *mainly if the condition develops while using an implant*
- Stroke, *mainly if the condition develops while using an implant*
- Breast cancer: can use if past history with no evidence of current disease for at least 5 years
- Active viral hepatitis
- Severe (decompensated) liver cirrhosis
- Liver tumours (benign and malignant)

Broadly usable with these conditions

- Before age 16 (theoretical concerns about hypo-oestrogenic effects)
- Questionable fertility from whatever reason
- Blood pressure equal or above 180/110mm Hg, or hypertension with vascular disease
- Diabetes with nephropathy/retinopathy/ neuropathy/other vascular disease, or duration of more than 20 years without vascular disease
- Current and history of ischaemic heart disease
- Stroke
- Known hyperlipidaemias
- Severe, recurrent headaches, including migraine with or without focal neurological symptoms
- Abnormal vaginal bleeding patterns: irregular without heavy bleeding, or with heavy or prolonged bleeding (including regular patterns)
- Cervical intraepithelial neoplasia (CIN) or cervical cancer awaiting treatment
- History of COC-related cholestasis
- Mild (compensated) liver cirrhosis
- Use of drugs which affect (induce) liver enzymes: rifampicin, rifabutin, griseofulvin, phenytoin, carbamazepine, barbiturates, primidone, topiramate, ritonavir

Initial assessment prior to insertion

A careful personal and family medical history with particular attention to cardiovascular risk factors, and an accurate blood pressure measurement is sufficient for most women. Further assessment is needed only if a relevant personal or family history is disclosed, or the blood pressure is very severely elevated. Routine screening by means of physical examination (including breast and bimanual pelvic examination), urine or blood tests should not be a pre-requisite before inserting an implant. Indeed, the routine use of such procedures can restrict accessibility to use of an implant, as well as other methods of contraception.

Monitoring during usage

The follow-up assessment should enquire about any problems, especially the development of new or more severe headaches and an assessment of any abnormal bleeding patterns.

levonorgestrel-releasing intrauterine system (IUS)

Description

T shaped plastic device which releases a small daily dose of levonorgestrel (about a third of that of a POP) from its polydimethylsiloxane reservoir through a rate limiting membrane for at least 5 years. Main effects are local: endometrial suppression, changes to cervical mucus and uterotubal fluid

Advantages

CONTRACEPTIVE

- Highly effective, non-intercourse related, rapidly reversible
- Can often be used by women with conditions which preclude the use of COCs, such as a history of venous thrombosis
- Immediately effective
- Does not interfere with breast-feeding

NON-CONTRACEPTIVE

- Reduced blood loss, sometimes amenorrhoea (after several months usage), modest rises in haemoglobin levels
- Less dysmenorrhoea
- Possibly reduced risk of clinical pelvic inflammatory disease
- Possibly reduced risk of extra-uterine pregnancies (because of its great efficiency at reducing all pregnancies whatever their site)

Disadvantages

- Expulsion (risk of pregnancy)
- Uterine or cervical perforation (highly dependent on the service provider, can result in risk of pregnancy; risk of bowel/bladder adhesions)
- Infection (greatest risk in first 20 days after insertion, probably related to pre-existing carriage of infection, before reverting to background risk of STIs)
- Hormonal side effects in first few months after insertion, including irregular, usually

light, uterine bleeding, increased duration of vaginal bleeding and functional ovarian cysts
- No research to show is effective as postcoital contraceptive, and therefore cannot be recommended for this purpose especially since it may be slightly slower to take effect than the copper IUD

Do not use with these conditions
- Pregnancy
- Post-septic abortion
- Unexplained vaginal bleeding (important to exclude serious underlying illness, especially before inserting IUS)
- Current breast cancer, if develops while using the IUS
- Pelvic inflammatory disease – current or within last 3 months, including purulent cervicitis
- Past episode or at high risk (eg heart valve prosthesis) of bacterial endocarditis
- Allergy to levonorgestrel
- Malignant gestational trophoblastic disease
- Severely distorted uterine cavity, cavity less than 5.5mm
- Strong immunosuppression (but standard regimens of corticosteroids are not a risk)

Use cautiously with these conditions
- Less than 4 weeks postpartum (because of concerns about perforation especially if breast-feeding, effects on uterine involution) NB. more usual time of insertion is about 6 weeks post-partum if woman had a vaginal delivery, 8 weeks if she had a Caesarian section
- Increased risk of STIs
- Active viral hepatitis
- Severe (decompensated) liver cirrhosis
- Benign and malignant liver tumours
- Benign gestational trophoblastic disease while human chorionic gonadotrophin (hCG) levels elevated ie currently active

Broadly usable with these conditions
- Second trimester abortion (because of concerns about increased risk of expulsion)
- Age less than 20 (concerns about risk of expulsion because of nulliparity)
- Diabetes with or without nephropathy/ retinopathy/neuropathy/other vascular disease or duration more than 20 years
- Current and history of ischaemic heart disease
- Stroke
- Known hyperlipidaemias
- Complicated valvular heart disease (unless associated with past endocarditis) [note: needs antibiotic cover at insertion]
- Abnormal vaginal bleeding patterns: with heavy or prolonged bleeding (including regular patterns), if condition develops while using an IUS
- Current breast cancer, if known about before insertion IUS; past history and no evidence of current disease for at least 5 years
- Past history of pelvic inflammatory disease (PID) (assuming no known current risk factors for STIs) without subsequent pregnancy
- Vaginitis without purulent cervicitis
- HIV positive
- Past COC-related cholestasis
- Mild (compensated) liver cirrhosis
- Uterine fibroids not distorting uterine cavity
- Nulliparity (concern arises because IUDs in such women may increase the risk of infection and expulsion)
- Anatomical abnormalities interfering with IUS insertion, such as cervical stenosis or cervical lacerations.
- Questionable fertility for whatever reason

NB. Many of the concerns mentioned above reflect the current lack of information about the effects of the progestogen provided by the system. The daily dosage, however, is less than the daily dose of POP. Many concerns, therefore, are theoretical rather than proven. Indeed the system may be particularly useful for some women with some of the above conditions if alternative contraceptives are unsatisfactory.

Initial assessment prior to insertion
A careful personal medical history with particular attention to gynaecological history and risk factors for STIs is required. Ideally all women should be screened for STIs, particularly Chlamydia trachomatis before insertion. Blind treatment with broad-spectrum antibiotics is a second best option as the opportunity for contact tracing is lost, thereby increasing the risk of rapid reinfection.

Monitoring during usage

The follow-up assessment should enquire about any problems, especially pain and bleeding. Either symptom should be assumed to be due to one the complications (infection, ectopic pregnancy, miscarriage, malposition), and excluded from the differential diagnosis before attributing them as side effects of the IUS. Examination (at 6-8 weeks, then at a minimum, annually), should check for partial expulsion/malposition and pelvic tenderness.

copper-bearing intrauterine devices (IUDs)

Description

Intrauterine device of copper wire curved round different shaped pieces of plastic or crimped to a polypropylene thread (GyneFix). Main effects: prevents fertilisation and blocks endometrial implantation.

Advantages

- Highly effective, non-intercourse related contraceptive
- Can often be used by women with conditions which preclude the use of COCs, such as a history of venous thrombosis
- Immediately effective
- Useful for postcoital contraception
- Does not interfere with breast-feeding

Disadvantages

- Intra-uterine pregnancy (miscarriage risk)
- Extra-uterine pregnancy (although the absolute risk of pregnancy is reduced, the fewer pregnancies which occur are more likely to be ectopic)
- Expulsion (risk of pregnancy)
- Uterine or cervical perforation (highly dependent on the service provider, can result in risk of pregnancy; risk of bowel/bladder adhesions)
- Infection (greatest risk in first 20 days after insertion, probably related to pre-existing carriage of infection, before reverting to background risk of STI)
- Pain (except GyneFix)
- Vaginal bleeding (increased amount/duration)

Do not use with these conditions

- Pregnancy
- Post-septic abortion
- Unexplained vaginal bleeding (important to exclude serious underlying illness, especially before inserting IUD)
- PID – current or within last 3 months, Including purulent cervicitis
- Known allergy to copper
- Wilson's Disease
- Malignant gestational trophoblastic disease
- Severely distorted uterine cavity, or cavity less than 5.5mm
- Past episode or at high risk (eg heart valve prosthesis) of bacterial endocarditis
- Strong immunosuppression (but standard regimens of corticosteroids are not a risk)

Use cautiously with these conditions

- 48 hours to 4 weeks postpartum (because of concerns about perforation, especially if breast-feeding). NB. More usual time of insertion is about 6 weeks postpartum if woman had a vaginal delivery, 8 weeks if she had a Caesarian section
- Increased risk of PID
- HIV positive, high risk of HIV, AIDS
- Benign gestational trophoblastic disease
- Past ectopic pregnancy in nulliparous woman (better to use an anovulant method)

Broadly usable with these conditions

- Less than 48 hours postpartum (because of concerns of increased risk of expulsion)
- Second trimester abortion (because of concerns about increased risk of expulsion)
- Age less than 20 (concerns about risk of expulsion because of nulliparity)
- Complicated valvular heart disease (do not use if associated with past endocarditis). NB. Needs antibiotic cover at insertion
- Abnormal vaginal bleeding patterns: with heavy or prolonged bleeding (including regular patterns)
- Cervical cancer awaiting treatment, if IUD already inserted
- Endometrial, ovarian cancer, if IUD already inserted

- Past history of PID (assuming no known current risk factors for STIs) without subsequent pregnancy
- Vaginitis without purulent cervicitis
- Uterine fibroids if not distorting uterine cavity
- Any severe anaemia: eg thalassaemia, sickle cell disease, iron deficiency anaemia
- Nulliparity (concern about increased risk of infection and exclusion)
- Anatomical abnormalities interfering with IUD insertion, such as cervical stenosis or cervical lacerations.
- Severe dysmenorrhoea
- Endometriosis
- Questionable fertility for whatever reason

Initial assessment prior to insertion

A careful personal medical history with particular attention to gynaecological history and risk factors for STIs is required. Ideally all women should be screened for STIs, particularly Chlamydia trachomatis before insertion. Blind treatment with broad-spectrum antibiotics is a second best option as the opportunity for contact tracing is lost, thereby increasing the risk of reinfection.

Monitoring during usage

The follow-up assessment should enquire about any problems, especially pain and bleeding. Either symptom should be assumed to be due to one the complications (infection, ectopic pregnancy, miscarriage, malposition), and excluded from the differential diagnosis before attributing them as side effects of the IUD. Examination (at 6-8 weeks, then at a minimum, annually), should check for partial expulsion/malposition and pelvic tenderness.

combined oral contraceptives (COCs)

Description

Combination of oestrogen and progestogen to prevent ovulation

Advantages

CONTRACEPTIVE

Highly effective, non-intercourse related, reversible

NON-CONTRACEPTIVE

- Reduced risk of ovarian and endometrial cancer, protection which increases with duration of use and persists for many years after cessation of COC use
- Reduction of most disorders of menstruation
- Users less likely to develop iron deficiency anaemia
- Fewer functional ovarian cysts
- Fewer extrauterine pregnancies because normal ovulation inhibited
- Reduced risk of PID
- Reduced risk of benign breast disease
- Probable reduction in rate of endometriosis
- Fewer symptomatic fibroids
- Probable reduction in thyroid disease (both overactive and underactive syndromes)
- Possible reduction in risk of rheumatoid arthritis
- Fewer sebaceous disorders (with oestrogen-dominant COCs)
- Possibly fewer duodenal ulcers (not well established and perhaps due to avoidance of COCs by women who are prone to anxiety)
- Reduction in Trichomonas vaginalis infections
- Possible lower incidence of toxic-shock syndrome

NB. Most of the evidence for the non-contraceptive benefits comes from studies of women using COCs with higher doses of hormones than currently used. Some of the benefits, therefore, may be smaller with currently available products, although limited evidence suggests that the benefits may be maintained.

Disadvantages

- Requires consistent regular use
- Increased risk of venous thromboembolic disease
- Increased risk of arterial disease (myocardial infarction, stroke, peripheral vascular disease) in COC users who smoke, or with other risk factors, and older women
- Increases in blood pressure which usually

reverse when COCs are stopped

- Possible increase in risk of localised breast cancer being diagnosed while using COCs and for up to ten years after stopping, *but less clinically advanced disease* (the relative risk is unaffected by a family history of breast cancer or personal history of benign breast disease, although both factors increase the risk of breast cancer so the absolute/ attributable risk is increased)
- Possible increase in risk of cervical cancer in long-term users
- Possible increase in risk of liver tumours, mainly in long-term users (very rare in British women)
- Possible increased risk of choriocarcinoma in women given COCs in the presence of active trophoblastic disease (hence advice in the UK to avoid using COCs while hCG levels are elevated)
- Often associated with a long list of non-bleeding, so-called 'minor', side effects, such as nausea, weight gain, bloatedness, breast tenderness, lassitude, acne, depression, many of which have not been substantiated by good clinical trial data

NB. There is still insufficient evidence to tell whether the overall cardiovascular risks associated with COCs have decreased as the hormonal content has declined, although there are some indications that they might have done. Furthermore, it is crucial to recognise that the incidence of all of the conditions mentioned above is very low at the age when most women use COCs (below 35 years). The absolute number of women affected will therefore be very small. For some conditions, this very low risk might be reduced further by a careful assessment before prescribing COCs.

Do not use with these conditions

- Pregnancy
- Unexplained vaginal bleeding (important to exclude serious abnormalities especially before initiating COC use)
- Breast-feeding, less than 6 weeks postpartum
- Blood pressure greater than 160/100 mm Hg
- Arterial disease, including ischaemic heart disease and stroke
- Deep venous, or other definite, thrombosis, or known high risk of this condition (congential or acquired thrombophilias)
- Complicated valvular heart disease, significant atrial or ventricle septal defect, pulmonary hypertension
- Severe recurrent migraine headaches, including those with focal neurological symptoms[3,9]
- Active trophoblastic disease (until hCG levels have returned to normal)
- Current breast, gynaecological or liver cancer
- Active hepatitis
- Severe (decompensated) liver cirrhosis
- Hepatic porphyria
- Major surgery with prolonged immobilisation, surgery to legs, prolonged immobilisation after fractures (temporary risk)

Use cautiously with these conditions

- Breast-feeding 6 weeks to 6 months postpartum (when main source of nutrition)
- Less than 3 weeks postpartum in non-breast-feeding woman
- Multiple risk factors for arterial disease, eg smoker *and* 35+ years
- Moderately raised blood pressure (140-159/90-99mm Hg), especially with other risk factors for arterial disease
- Diabetes *with* nephropathy/retinopathy/ neuropathy/other vascular disease or diabetes of more than 20 years' duration
- Known hyperlipidaemias, especially if severe or with other risk factors for arterial disease
- Past breast or cervical cancer with no evidence of current disease for at least 5 years
- Medically treated or current biliary tract disease
- Past history of COC-related cholestasis
- Mild (compensated) liver cirrhosis
- Use of drugs which affect (induce) liver enzymes: rifampicin, rifabutin, griseofulvin, phenytoin, carbamazepine, barbiturates, primidone, topiramate, ritonavir). See below

Broadly usable with these conditions

- Breast-feeding more than 6 months postpartum (when main source of nutrition)
- Aged more than 35 years, if other risk factors

for arterial disease (especially smoking) are absent
- Aged less than 35 years *and* a smoker (regular encouragement to stop smoking – rather than stop COC use – is needed)
- Diabetes without vascular disease
- Superficial thrombophlebitis
- Known hyperlipidaemias, if mild and no other risk factors for arterial disease
- Uncomplicated mild valvular heart disease
- Recurrent headaches, including migraine without focal neurological symptoms (these become an unacceptable risk if more than once a month and are associated with other significant arterial risk factors, including age over 35)[3,9]
- Cervical intraepithelial neoplasia (CIN) or cervical cancer awaiting treatment
- Symptomatic biliary tract disease treated by cholecystectomy
- History of pregnancy related cholestasis
- Sickle cell disease (but *not* sickle cell trait which is not a problem)
- Major surgery without prolonged immobilisation (temporary risk)

Initial assessment prior to COC use

It will be apparent that most of the conditions given above are rare in young women. A careful personal and family medical history with particular attention to cardiovascular risk factors, and an accurate blood pressure measurement is sufficient for most women[2]. Further assessment is needed only if a relevant personal or family history is disclosed, or the blood pressure is elevated. Routine screening by means of physical examination (including breast and bimanual pelvic examination), urine or blood tests should not be a pre-requisite for obtaining COCs. Indeed, the routine use of such procedures can restrict accessibility to use of COCs, as well as other methods of contraception.

Monitoring during usage

The follow-up assessment should:
- enquire about any new risk factors which might have developed
- ask about any symptoms, especially headaches
- check that the pill is being taken correctly
- check the blood pressure

There is no consensus about how frequently the blood pressure needs to be taken. Many practitioners would check it initially after 1-3 months of use, then 6 monthly, with perhaps an extension of the interval to annual checks if the blood pressure remains low after 2 or 3 years of use. There is no need for other screening procedures simply because a woman is using COCs.

Starting the pill

The first pill visit covers a lot of ground and it is important to make sure that the following is given:
- written up-to-date information about COCs, such as the FPA leaflet *Choosing and using the combined pill* (latest edition), for the woman to read and keep for future reference, with specific details of issues relating to everyday (ED) pills if prescribed
- advice that each new pack of pills should be started on the same day of the week
- information that even if bleeding occurs while taking the pill, the pack should be finished
- advice that intercourse during the pill-free interval is only safe if the next pack is used on time; otherwise alternative contraceptives are required from the last pill in the pack
- information that even if bleeding has not stopped, the next pack should be started on time
- advice about what to do with missed pills, if vomiting occurs or tablets which interfere with COCs are taken (give written advice)
- when to seek advice immediately
- who is available in the practice to give advice

Missed COCs

Accepted guidelines regarding missed combined pills are:

A combined pill is regarded as 'missed' if it is taken more than 12 hours late. If it is remembered within 12 hours, contraceptive protection is not lost. The missed pill should be taken as soon as it is remembered. The next pill should be taken at the normal time. This may mean more than one pill is taken in one day. If more than one pill is missed, the last missed pill should be taken and the rest of the packet taken at the usual time. An extra contraceptive method must be used for 7 days. If the missed pill occurred during the last week of the packet, the pack should be finished, and a new packet should be started immediately thereby eliminating the pill-free interval. With ED pills, the 7 days of using an additional contraceptive method must include active pills to ensure contraceptive cover; this means ensuring that non-active (placebo) tablets are missed out[4].

Postcoital contraception (see Part 6) is only indicated if the pill-free (ie contraception-free) time has been increased to 9 days, or the pills missed have led to an equivalent duration free of the pill's actions[3,10]

Concomitant use of other drugs

LONG TERM USE OF LIVER ENZYME INDUCING DRUGS

Anti-infectives (rifampicin, rifabutin and griseofulvin) and anticonvulsants (phenytoin, carbamazepine, barbiturates, primidone, topiramate and ritonavir) require consideration of whether an alternative method of contraception is needed. Otherwise there should be an increase in COC dose with a shortening, or possible elimination, of the pill-free interval (eg 'tricycling'[3,4,5]).

SHORT TERM USE OF LIVER ENZYME INDUCING DRUGS OR BROAD SPECTRUM ANTIBIOTICS

Ampicillin, amoxycillin, augmentin, tetracyclines, broad spectrum cephalosporins require extra precautions during treatment and for a further 7 days after stopping. This may require the elimination of the next pill-free interval if the last potentially less effective pill was taken during the last week of the pack. Rifampicin is such a powerful enzyme inducer that even if taken for only 2 days (eg to eliminate carriage of meningococcus) increased elimination of COC must be assumed for 4 weeks thereafter.

NB. Co-trimoxazole and erythromycin do not affect contraceptive cover – if anything they increase the blood levels of ethinyloestradiol, but not dangerously so.

LONG-TERM USE OF BROAD-SPECTRUM ANTIBIOTICS

Within about 2 weeks the large bowel flora responsible for recycling oestrogen have reconstituted with resistant organisms. Thus, extra precautions are no longer needed after 2 weeks.

OTHER DRUGS

Occasional reports have appeared suggesting that COCs influence the pharmacotherapeutic effect of other drugs (eg analgesics, antidepressants, antimalarial drugs, benzodiazepines, B-blockers, corticosteroids, hypoglycaemic drugs, oral anticoagulants and theophylline). The documentation level regarding these interactions varies from 'possible' to 'probable'. So far, however, there is no evidence to suggest clinically significant effects which require the adjustment of the dose or prescription of an alternative medication[11].

progestogen only pills (POPs)

Description

Daily dose of oral progestogen which works primarily by making the cervical mucus hostile to sperm penetration, but may also prevent ovulation in some cycles, and has endometrial effects

Advantages

- Effective, non-intercourse related, reversible
- Can often be used by women with conditions which preclude the use of COCs such as history of venous thromboembolism
- Does not interfere with breast-feeding

Disadvantages

- Requires consistent use every day, therefore not useful for forgetful users
- Menstrual irregularity, from amenorrhoea to

heavier more frequent periods; unpredictable and variable even in long-term users

- Breast tenderness, often transient
- Effect may be diminished in large or heavy women (arbitrarily defined as over 70 kg) (the evidence is uncertain, but this should be discussed with the woman and dose doubled if risk of pregnancy unacceptable)
- Hormonal contraceptives containing progestogen-only have not been widely used, but the pattern of risk of breast cancer with time since last use is similar to that found for COCs[8]

Do not use with these conditions

- Pregnancy
- Current breast cancer, *mainly if condition develops while using a POP*
- Allergy to hormone in the POP

Use cautiously with these conditions

- Current and history of ischaemic heart disease, *mainly if the condition develops while using a POP*
- Stroke, *mainly if the condition develops while using a POP*
- Breast cancer: current at time of considering starting POP, or past history with no evidence of current disease for at least 5 years
- Choriocarcinoma (until hCG levels have returned to normal)
- Active viral hepatitis
- Severe (decompensated) liver cirrhosis
- Liver tumours (benign and malignant)
- Use of drugs which affect (induce) liver enzymes: rifampicin, rifabutin, griseofulvin, phenytoin, carbamazepine, barbiturates, primidone, topiramate, ritonavir (double dose if used)

Broadly usable with these conditions

- Age before age 16 (theoretical concerns about hypo-oestrogenic effects)
- Blood pressure equal or greater than 180/110mm Hg, or hypertension with vascular disease
- Diabetes with nephropathy/retinopathy/neuropathy/other vascular disease, or duration of more than 20 years without vascular disease
- Current and history of ischaemic heart disease
- Stroke
- Known hyperlipidaemias
- Severe, recurrent headaches, including migraine with focal neurological symptoms
- Abnormal vaginal bleeding patterns: irregular without heavy bleeding, or with heavy or prolonged bleeding (including regular patterns)
- Undiagnosed breast mass
- Cervical intraepithelial neoplasia (CIN) or cervical cancer awaiting treatment
- History of COC-related cholestasis
- Mild (compensated) liver cirrhosis
- Past ectopic pregnancy (POP use actually reduces the risk of ectopic pregnancy (because it prevents ovulation in many users), but other methods with more consistent suppression of ovulation (eg COC, DMPA) may be preferable)
- Functional cysts causing pain

Initial assessment prior to POP use

A careful personal and family medical history with particular attention to cardiovascular risk factors, and an accurate blood pressure measurement is sufficient for most women. Further assessment is needed only if a relevant personal or family history is disclosed, or the blood pressure is very severely elevated. Routine screening by means of physical examination (including breast and bimanual pelvic examination), urine or blood tests should not be a pre-requisite for obtaining POPs. Indeed, the routine use of such procedures can restrict accessibility to use of POPs, as well as other methods of contraception.

Monitoring during usage

The follow-up assessment should include enquiries about any problems. POPs do not appear to affect blood pressure in previously normotensive women, but may cause a small rise in women who have previously experienced blood pressure increases while using a COC. Given the simplicity and cheapness of the procedure, we recommend the monitoring of the blood pressure of a POP user annually.

Missed POPs

A POP is regarded as 'missed' if taken only 3 hours late. If this occurs the missed pill should be taken immediately and normal pill-taking resumed when the next pill is due. Additional contraceptive measures are needed for 7 days[4].

barrier methods

Description

Various devices of different materials used by women and men to provide a physical barrier between the ejaculate and the female genital tract. Efficiency can be increased by the simultaneous use of spermicides, especially with diaphragms and caps. Spermicides used alone are not usually recommended, although they may be sufficiently effective in women when fertility is decreased, eg during the climacteric.

Advantages

CONTRACEPTIVE

- Readily available
- Reasonable efficiency if used properly
- May be preferred by couples who have infrequent intercourse, especially those wishing to have a 'more natural' form of birth control
- Important adjunct when oral contraceptives are forgotten or of reduce efficacy (eg during use of some antibiotics)

NON-CONTRACEPTIVE

- Useful protection against STIs (especially condoms)
- Does not interfere with breast-feeding

Disadvantages

- Reliant on user for effectiveness, intercourse-related
- Often disliked because of aesthetics, reduced sensitivity during intercourse (with latex condoms)

Do not use with these conditions

- Any condition where pregnancy would be totally unacceptable to the user (use a more effective method)

Use cautiously with these conditions

- Irritation or sensitivity to latex (condoms/diaphragms are often made of latex: plastic condoms exist)
- History of toxic shock syndrome (diaphragm)

Broadly usable with these conditions

- Complicated valvular heart disease (diaphragm users: risk of urinary tract infection may increase risk of developing sub-acute bacterial endocarditis)
- Cervical cancer awaiting treatment (spermicide or cap not recommended)
- High risk HIV (repeated and/or high doses of spermicide may cause vaginal wall abrasions, increasing the risk of transmission)
- Parity (parous diaphragm users have a higher risk of failure than nulliparous users)
- Recurrent urinary tract infections in diaphragm users (use a smaller cervical cap instead)

natural family planning/fertility awareness

Description

Variety of methods to recognise or predict the timing of ovulation, in order to identify the fertile period:

- calender method
- temperature method
- cervical mucus method
- sympto-thermal/multiple index method
- fertility devices (eg Persona)

The sympto-thermal method is the most effective (80 to 98 per cent effective) because it combines more than one indicator of fertility. With all fertility awareness methods, including Persona, careful adherence to the guidelines is important to ensure success.

Women should be advised that the first (pre-ovulatory) phase of reduced fertility is less 'safe', *however identified*, than the second (post-ovulatory) phase; greater efficacy can be achieved by restricting unprotected intercourse to the latter phase.

Advantages

- No known physical side effects
- Non-intercourse related
- May be only acceptable contraceptive for some with religious or personal beliefs which prevent using other methods of birth control
- Once learnt does not need regular follow-up
- Can be used to plan pregnancy as well as prevent conception

Disadvantages

- Requires commitment from both partners
- For most success, teaching probably requires specialist knowledge from natural family planning teachers
- Requires careful observation and record keeping, with documentation of a number of cycles before ovulation can be reliably predicted
- Fertility devices (Persona) are expensive to buy and use

Breast-feeding (lactational amenorrhoea method–LAM)

Breast-feeding is a recognised effective contraceptive (98 per cent) provided that:

- the woman is fully or almost fully breast-feeding (ie using no milk substitutes and feeding on demand day and night), *and*
- the baby is less than six months old, *and*
- menstruation has not returned

As soon as any one of these conditions change, alternative methods of contraception should be started.

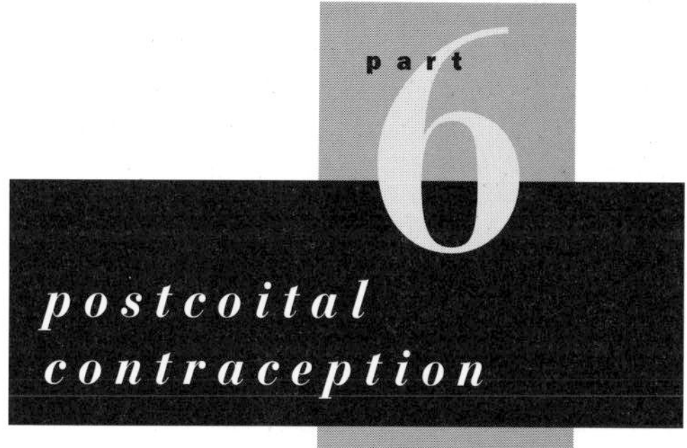

postcoital contraception

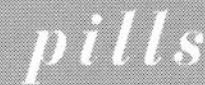

pills

Description

Two pills, each of 50 micrograms ethinyloestradiol with 250 micrograms levonorgestrel, repeated 12 hours later (Yupze method); first set of pills taken within 72 hours of first act of unprotected intercourse

Alternatively, several progestogen-only methods have been used, although most published studies have included small numbers of women[10]. As yet there is no licensed progestogen-only product for emergency contraception.

Advantages

- Highly effective contraceptive (95 per cent effective mid-cycle, 98 per cent at other times[12]
- Useful back-up for those who have had unprotected intercourse, including rape victims

Disadvantages

- High frequency of nausea with Yupze method, severe vomiting may compromise effectiveness. If desired, the Faculty of Family Planning and Reproductive Health Care recommends Domperidone (10mg) taken just before each dose

Do not use with these conditions

- Pregnancy
- Current hepatocellular jaundice (consider IUD)
- Sickle cell crisis (consider IUD)

Use cautiously with these conditions

- History of severe cardiovascular complications, angina pectoris, venous thromboembolism
- Focal migraine, with headache occurring at time of request for postcoital contraception NB. Many authorities would place the above in the 'do not use' section

Broadly usable with these conditions

Using an enzyme inducing drug (in which case increase dose COC/POP by 50 per cent or use IUD). No need to increase the dose for non enzyme inducing antibiotics

Initial assessment prior to use

The history should include details of the last menstrual period, length of menstrual cycle, timing of all inadequately protected intercourse in this cycle (to ensure that the *first* episode of unprotected intercourse occurred less than 72 hours previously), history of cardiovascular disease, including thromboembolism, focal migraine. The consultation is usually a useful opportunity to review continuing contraceptive needs and other aspects of sexual health. The blood pressure should usually be measured as part of good clinical practice, but other procedures are rarely indicated.

Women should be advised that their next period may be earlier or later than usual, or on time. A few women have light bleeding shortly after taking hormonal postcoital contraception, this is not the next period.

Monitoring after usage

The woman should be offered a follow-up appointment for 3 to 4 weeks, unless she develops lower abdominal pain, heavy bleeding, or she is concerned or worried, when she should be seen sooner. If the next menstrual period is abnormally light, short or absent pregnancy should be suspected and managed as any other unintended pregnancy, since the pregnancy would not have been exposed to the postcoital hormones which were given pre-implantation.

insertion of an IUD

Description

Insertion of copper IUD (ie not hormone releasing) up to 5 days after earliest ovulation, calculated from woman's shortest likely cycle

Advantages

- Most effective available method (2 failures in 1300 insertions[6])
- Offers continuing contraception, but if not appropriate can be removed at next menses
- Useful when hormonal postcoital contraception has induced vomiting and replacement dose not sufficient to provide adequate cover
- Useful if multiple exposure
- Useful if current focal migraine, jaundice, sickle cell crisis or history of cardiovascular disease

Disadvantages

- Pain
- Bleeding
- Risk of infection

Do not use with these conditions

- Pregnancy
- As for IUDs generally (see page 92)

Use cautiously with these conditions

- As for IUDs generally (see page 92)

Broadly usable with these conditions

- As for IUDs generally, except history of past ectopic pregnancies (see pages 92 and 93)

Initial assessment prior to insertion

The history should include details of the last menstrual period, length of menstrual cycle, timing of all inadequately protected intercourse in this cycle (to ensure that the insertion is within five days of ovulation) and aspects of history required to ensure the safe insertion of an IUD. The consultation is usually a useful opportunity to review continuing contraceptive needs and other aspects of sexual health. The blood pressure should usually be measured as part of good clinical practice. Ideally all women should be screened for STIs and antibiotic cover provided (see page 93).

Monitoring after usage

The woman should be offered a follow-up appointment for 3 to 4 weeks, unless she develops lower abdominal pain, heavy bleeding, or she is concerned or worried, when she should be seen sooner. If the next menstrual period is abnormally light, short or absent pregnancy should be suspected. It should be managed as any other unintended pregnancy, except if going to term the IUD should be removed to reduce the risk of miscarriage[4].

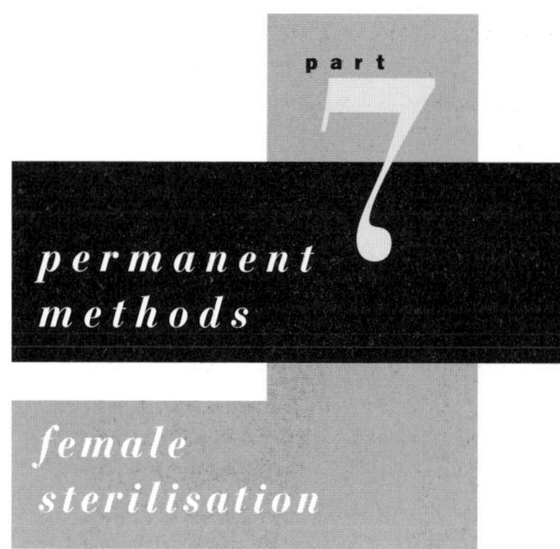

Description

Occlusion of the fallopian tubes by a variety of surgical techniques (most commonly, mechanical means such as tubal clips or rings; also diathermy or partial salpingectomy) using a variety of surgical approaches (most frequently laparoscopy, but also laparotomy or mini-laparotomy)

Advantages

- Highly effective
- Immediacy of effect
- Permanent
- Not reliant on the user for effect
- Can remove the fear of pregnancy

Disadvantages

- Requires a surgical procedure (usually under light general anaesthetic but can be under local anaesthetic)
- Sometimes fails (failure rate 1-5 per 1,000 – depends on method used; perhaps 25 to 50 per cent of the failures occur some years after the operation, emphasising the need to warn women to mention that they have been sterilised if they subsequently develop pelvic pain; failure is more common in younger women; perhaps a third of such pregnancies are ectopic)
- Not necessarily reversible (success of reversal more likely if clips rather than another method used, and if the woman is younger. Pregnancies after reversal are also more likely to be ectopic).

- Can cause regret (appears to be more common if done at young age (under 30 years), at time of relationship difficulties, if partnership is child-free, if performed just after childbirth, termination of pregnancy or miscarriage, when ambivalent about whether to have the operation).
- Has been said to cause menstrual upset afterwards although the evidence is inconsistent and may be due to other factors such as stopping COCs which were masking menstrual problems

Special precautions
In general, the medical precautions are those which exist for any woman requiring a light general anaesthetic. The operation may be technically more difficult in obese women (laparoscopic sterilisation) or certain gynaecological problems.

Initial assessment before the operation
Ideally both partners should be involved in the decision. Careful counselling is required about the operation's permanence, risk of failure (including risk of ectopic pregnancy), and reassurance about no clear evidence of adverse effect on menstrual pattern. Information that vasectomy is equally as effective, but quicker, safer and cheaper than female sterilisation, should also be given. The greater tendency for childless women, and those aged less than 30 years, to regret their decision, means that such women and their partners need particularly careful counselling. Contraceptive measures should be used up to the day of the procedure. In particular, there is no need for women using COCs to discontinue the pill beforehand.

Monitoring after operation
Apart from the usual post-operative care, no other measures are required. Signs of ectopic pregnancy should be sought if any periods are missed, light or scanty especially if associated with lower abdominal pain.

male sterilisation

Description
Excision of a segment, and occlusion by ligature, cautery or clip of remaining, vas deferentia by a small incision or puncture of the scrotal skin.

Advantages
- Highly effective
- Permanent
- Safe and easy, usually can be done under local anaesthesia
- Not reliant on the user for effect
- Can remove the fear of pregnancy

Disadvantages
- Not effective immediately (may take 3 to 4 months; clinics vary when they start testing for effect)
- Requires a surgical procedure
- Sometimes fails (failure rate about 1 per 1,000: can occur some years after operation even if the man had previously had negative sperm counts, chances of late failure 1 in 3,000 to 1 in 7,000)
- Not necessarily reversible (success of reversal depends on: method used; age of man (better in younger men); interval between sterilisation and reversal attempt (poor if more than 10 years))
- Can cause regret (appears to be more common if done at young age (under 30 years), if the partnership is child-free, if done at time of relationship difficulties, when ambivalent about whether to have the operation)
- Short term side effects of scrotal bruising and swelling (less with the 'no scalpel' technique)
- Sperm granuloma causing the formation of nodules can occur in up to 30 per cent of men after vasectomy; tenderness is rare and lesion rarely needs excision

Anti-sperm antibodies have been reported in a large proportion of men after vasectomy, but these do not appear to be associated with increased auto-immune disease. Previous concerns that vasectomy increases the risk of cardiovascular disease have not been substantiated. Some studies have indicated that vasectomy increases the risk of prostatic and testicular cancer; findings which have been contradicted by other researchers. On the basis of existing biological and epidemiological evidence, any causal relationship between vasectomy and risk of prostate and testicular cancer is unproven and no changes in family planning policies concerning vasectomy are justified. It is important, however, to include discussion of the subject as part of the counselling, if only because future research is likely to attract media attention.

Special precautions

In general, there are few medical precautions for the operation. The operation may be technically more difficult in men with certain urological problems.

Initial assessment before the operation

Ideally both partners should be involved in the decision. Careful counselling about the operation's permanence and risk of failure is required. The greater tendency for men who are childless, or aged less than 30 years, to regret their decision, means that such men and their partners need particularly careful counselling.

Monitoring after operation

Other contraceptive measures should be used until 2 consecutive negative semen samples have been obtained.

Table 1. Conditions requiring particular consideration when choosing a reversible method of contraception

	Progestogen injection (Inj)	Progestogen implant (Imp)	Intrauterine system (IUS)	Intrauterine device (IUD)	Combined oral contraceptive (COC)	Progestogen only pill (POP)	Barrier methods (Bar)
Age <16	❍	❍				❍	
<20			❍	❍			
Non-smoker >35					❍		
Smoker <35					❍		
>35					◗		
Nulliparity			❍	❍			
Parity							❍
Pregnant	●	●	●	●	●	●	
Questionable fertility from whatever reason	❍	❍	❍	❍			
Post-partum, almost exclusive breast-feeding: <6 weeks	◗	◗	◗	◗	●		
6 weeks to 6 months					◗		
>6 months					❍		
Post-partum, not breast-feeding almost exclusively: <48 hours			◗	❍	◗		
48 hours to 4 weeks			◗	◗	◗		
Post-abortion: 2nd trimester			❍	❍			
septic abortion			●	●			
Past ectopic pregnancy in nulliparous women				◗		❍	
Trophoblastic disease: malignant			●	●	●		
benign			❍a	❍a	❍a	❍a	
Diabetes (insulin and non-insulin dependent): without vascular problems	❍		❍		❍		
with vascular problems or >20 years duration	◗	❍	❍		◗	❍	
Hypertension: without vascular problems: 140-159/90-99mm Hg	❍				◗		
160-179/100-109mm Hg	❍				●		
180+/110+mm Hg	◗	❍			●	❍	
with vascular problems	◗	❍			●	❍	
Ischaemic heart disease: current/personal history	◗	◗b/ ❍c	❍		●	◗b/ ❍c	
Structural heart disease: uncomplicated valvular					❍		
complicated valvular			❍	❍	●		❍
significant atrial or ventricular septal effect					●		
Bacterial endocarditis: past episode or high risk			●	●			
Stroke: current/personal history	◗	◗b/ ❍c	❍		●	◗b/ ❍c	
Deep vein thrombosis/pulmonary embolus:							
current/personal history					●		
known high risk (congenital or acquired thrombophilia					●		
prolonged immobilisation (eg major surgery, leg fractures)					●		
major surgery without prolonged immobilisation					❍		
Superficial thrombosis					❍		
Known hyperlipidaemia	❍	❍	❍		◗b/ ❍c	❍	
Headaches: severe, recurrent including migraine without focal symptoms		❍			❍		
severe, recurrent including migraine with focal symptoms		❍			●	❍	
Breast disease: cancer – current	●	●	●b/ ❍c		●	●b /◗c	
cancer – past and no evidence of disease for 5 years	◗	◗	❍		◗	◗	

	Inj (Progestogen injection)	Imp (Progestogen implant)	IUS (Intrauterine system)	IUD (Intrauterine device)	COC (Combined oral contraceptive)	POP (Progestogen only pill)	Bar (Barrier methods)
Vaginal bleeding: unexplained	●	●	●	●	●		
irregular without heavy loss	❍	❍				❍	
heavy/prolonged loss (+/– irregular)	❍	❍	❍b	❍		❍	
with severe dysmenorrhoea				❍			
Carcinoma-in-situ of cervix		❍d			❍d	❍d	
Cervical cancer		❍d			●/ ◗e	❍d	❍d
Ovarian: cancer					●		
functional cysts causing pain						❍	
Endometrial cancer			●c	●cd/ ❍bd	●		
Uterine fibroids distorting the uterine cavity			❍	❍			
Anatomic abnormalities: severely distorting uterine cavity, <5.5mm size			●	●			
interfering with insertion, eg cervical stenosis			❍	❍			
Endometriosis				❍			
Pelvic inflammatory disease: past without subsequent pregnancy			❍	❍			
current or within 3 months			●	●			
increased risk				◗			
Sexually transmitted infection: current or within 3 months			●	●			
vaginitis without purulent cervicitis			❍	❍			
increased risk			◗	◗			
HIV/AIDS: HIV +ve			❍	◗			
high risk HIV/AIDS			◗	◗			❍
Toxic shock syndrome: past history							◗
Urinary tract infection: recurrent							❍
Biliary tract disease: symptomatic					◗		
Cholestasis: pregnancy-related					❍		
past combined oral contraceptive-related	❍	❍	❍		◗	❍	
Viral hepatitis: active	◗	◗	◗		●	◗	
Liver cirrhosis: mild	❍	❍	❍		◗	❍	
severe	◗	◗	◗		●	◗	
Hepatic porphrias					●		
Wilson's disease				●			
Liver tumours: benign + malignant	◗	◗	◗		●	◗	
Thalassaemia				❍			
Sickle cell *disease* (not trait – which is unaffected by choice)				❍	❍		
Iron deficiency anaemia				❍			
Allergy to: levonorgestrel		●	●			●	
copper				●			
latex							◗
Drug interactions – liver enzyme inducers:							
anti-infectives (rifampicin, rifabutin, griseofulvin)	❍	❍			◗	◗	
anti-convulsants (phenytoin, carbamezepine, barbiturates, primidone, topiramate, ritonavir)	❍	❍			◗	◗	
Strong immunosuppressive (but corticosteroids alright)			●	●			

● do not use with these conditions
◗ use cautiously with these conditions
❍ broadly usable with these conditions
a only while hCG levels elevated; not contra-indicated once hCG levels return to normal
b if develops during usage
c if known about at time of considering starting
d awaiting treatment
e past disease
Note: antineoplastic treatment may render women sterile

Table 2. Efficacy of contraceptive methods

Methods that have no 'user' failure	% per 100 women per year
Injectable contraception	over 99% effective
Intrauterine system (IUS)	over 99% effective in first year (over 98% over five years)
Intrauterine device (IUD)	over 99% effective (depending on IUD type)
Female sterilisation	over 99% effective, failure rate of 1-5 per 1,000 depending on method used
Male sterilisation (vasectomy)	over 99% effective, failure rate of about 1 per 1,000 (chance of late failure after 2 negative sperm counts – 1 in 3,000 to 1 in 7,000)
Methods that have 'user' failure	
Combined oral contraceptive	up to 99+% effective
Progestogen-only oral contraceptive	up to 99% effective
Male condom	up to 98% effective
Female condom	up to 95% effective
Diaphragm or cap + spermicide	up to 96% effective
Natural family planning:	
sympto-thermal method	up to 98% effective
new technologies (Persona)	up to 94% effective

NB. Efficacy rates of methods with 'user' failure reflect the method being used absolutely correctly and consistently. Where methods are used less well, lower efficacy will be seen.

Reproduced from the *FPA Contraceptive Handbook*[4]

Table 3. Risks of pregnancy with no contraception

Age of woman (years)	% per 100 women per year
<40	80–90%
40	40–50%
45	10–20%
50+	0–5%

Figures from *Contraception Today*[3]

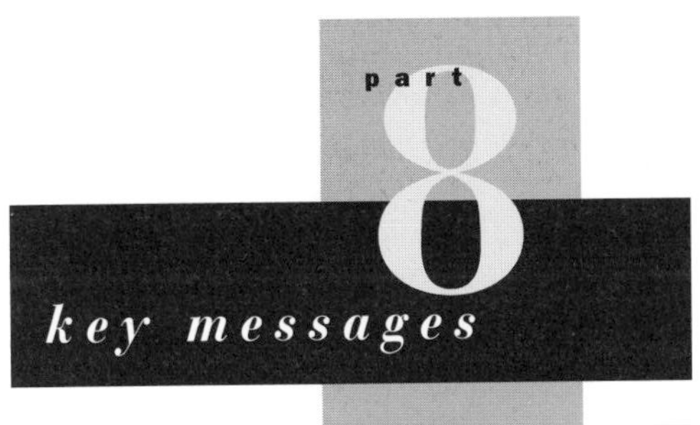

- The primary care team has the opportunity to provide high quality contraceptive services
- Decisions about the choice of contraceptive involve a number of issues including method effectiveness, perceived safety, recognised contraindications, acceptability, ease of use, and availability
- Users of contraceptive services need up-to-date comprehensive information about each method of contraception
- The primary care team need to ensure that the full range of contraceptive methods are available, even if this requires referral to another agency
- In the end, confidence in the services provided depends on the provision and standard of care
- Confident contraceptive users are more likely to use their chosen method of fertility regulation successfully

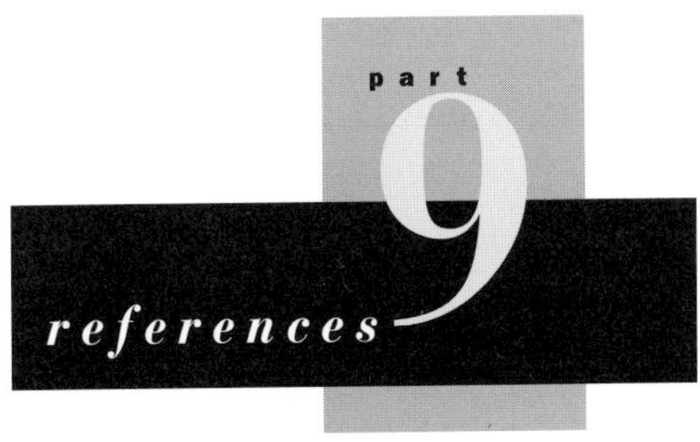

1 ***Improving access to quality care in family planning*: medical eligibility criteria for contraceptive use,** World Health Organization, Geneva, 1996

2 'Evidence-guided prescribing of combined oral contraceptives: consensus statement', Hannaford PC and Webb AMC on behalf of participants at an international workshop, ***Contraception, 54***, 1996, 125-29

3 ***Contraception today,*** Guillebaud J, Martin Dunitz, 1997

4 ***FPA contraceptive handbook,*** Belfield T, 2nd edn, Family Planning Association, 1997

5 ***Contraception – your questions answered,*** Guillebaud J, Churchill Livingstone, 1994

6 ***Handbook of family planning and reproductive health care,*** Loudon N, Glaiser A and Gebbie A (eds), Churchill Livingstone, 1995

7 'Contraceptive failure in the United States: an update', Trussell J, Hatcher RA and Cates W, et al, ***Studies in Family Planning, 21,*** 1990, 51-54

8 'Breast cancer and hormonal contraceptives: further results', Collaborative Group on Hormonal Factors in Breast Cancer, ***Contraception, 54*** (suppl), 1996, 1-106S

9 'Combined oral contraceptives, migraine and ischaemic stroke - joint recommendations from the Faculty of Family Planning and the Family Planning Association', ***British Journal of Family Planning, 1997*** (in press)

10 ***Emergency contraception guidelines for doctors,*** Kubba A, Faculty of Family Planning and Reproductive Health Care, 1995

11 ***Summary of drug interactions with oral contraceptives,*** Geurts TBP, Goorissen EM and Sitsen JMA, et al, Parthenon Publishing Group, 1993

12 'The efficacy of postcoital hormonal contraception', Trussell J and Stewart F, ***Family Planning Perspectives, 24, 1992,*** 262–64

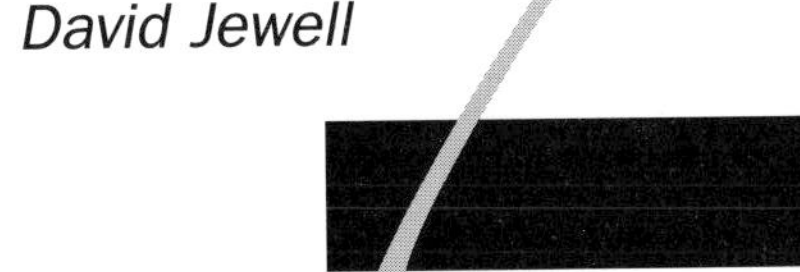

David Jewell

chapter seven

optimising pregnancy outcome and preconception care

part I
the attraction of preconception care

Preconception care is a beguiling idea, and the reasoning behind it obvious. Once effective contraceptive services are widely available planned pregnancy becomes possible. For many years certain factors in women's family, personal, medical and obstetric histories have been recognised as affecting the outcome of pregnancy. Taken together these elements lead directly to the notion of preconception care: by counselling women even before they become pregnant they will be helped to achieve better outcomes for pregnancy.

Using the model of primary, secondary and tertiary prevention, antenatal care might be compared to tertiary prevention, providing care to minimise the risks once pregnancy has started. Preconception care, by offering help before the event, could be compared to primary prevention. Unfortunately the story of medical intervention in pregnancy is littered with examples of the professionals and technology offering rather more than they have been able to deliver[1]. Such examples include fetal movement counting and routine antenatal cardiotocography, neither of which has been shown to improve fetal outcomes. Above all there is the example from intrapartum care of electronic fetal monitoring which by general consensus increases the risk of Caesarean section without improving the long term fetal outcome (the risk of neonatal fits is reduced but they are not associated with long term neurological problems). Armed with such knowledge it is vital to make sure that enthusiasm for an attractive idea doesn't lure primary care teams into the same trap where preconception care is concerned.

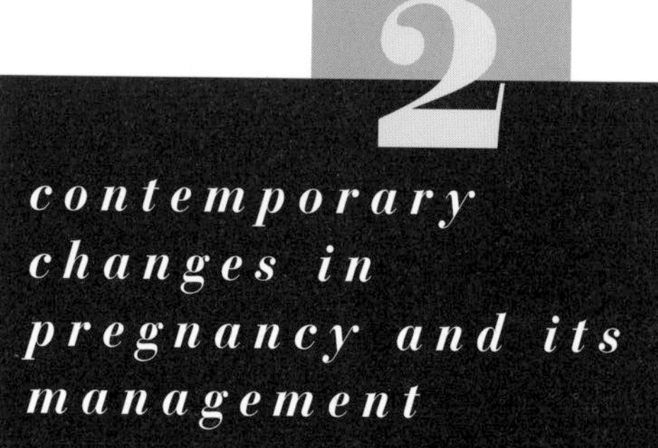

part 2
contemporary changes in pregnancy and its management

The whole approach to the way in which pregnancy is seen by patients and carers is changing. There is a move towards a less regimented approach to antenatal and intranatal care.

The *Changing childbirth* report[2] explicitly acknowledged that women's own views are important. In many cases there are no clear answers as to the most effective management of given clinical problems, at least not in isolation from women's personal feelings and beliefs. *Changing childbirth* has called for more 'woman-centred care' implying the desire to involve women more in decisions concerning their own care. Many reasons have been suggested to explain such changes. For some it is the result of a change in the balance of power between men and women, and reflects the way that midwives have collectively taken on more autonomous responsibility for pregnancy, as well as improving their own status in relation to obstetricians. Or it may be a reflection of a more widespread loss of automatic respect for authority figures. Also, over the last 20 years or so, there has been a changing attitude towards health promotion that concentrates more heavily on individuals taking steps to lead a 'more healthy lifestyle' and less on collective actions being taken to improve institutional causes of ill-health. Finally the growth of modern genetics has brought with it the prospect of being able to identify antenatally a wide range of congenital problems, introducing ethical, as well as practical, difficulties[3,4].

part 3 a broader approach: optimising pregnancy outcome

There is a tendency among medical professionals to take a narrow view of what constitutes health promotion. Many doctors tend to equate it with prevention, seeing it as activities which are undertaken as part of organised programmes of primary, secondary and tertiary prevention.

But it is possible to take a broader, more flexible view of health promotion which involves making the most of the opportunities that life presents. Health promotion would then comprise anything that assists such changes. It would include very simple actions on the part of professionals such as imparting information on health matters to enable patients to make choices about their own health.

Preconception care can be defined as any programmes or services undertaken before or around the time of conception that improve the outcome of pregnancy. It encompasses a wide range of activity occurring at different times in both women's and men's lives. Most importantly, this includes the provision of health and sex education in schools, and the provision of freely available contraceptive services, both of which should enable women and men to control both the number and timing of their pregnancies. The efforts currently being made to reduce the pregnancy rate among teenagers could be seen to be directed to the same end. More controversial, but nevertheless within this more widely defined scope of preconception advice, is the argument that reduction of socioeconomic differentials would improve pregnancy outcomes overall more than any other single intervention[5].

It also includes certain actions taken in one pregnancy to improve the outcome in the next one. The most obvious example here is postnatal administration of Anti D antibody to those women who are at risk of being sensitised by rhesus positive babies. This cannot be said to benefit the current pregnancy, but has played a huge part in improving the outcome in subsequent ones. In the same way, but with more mixed effects, one can see efforts to reduce the Caesarean section rate as important, not just in its effects on the index pregnancy, but also on the effect it has on choices that are available to women in subsequent ones.

Fig 1

not sexually active	sexually active, not pregnant	pregnant	post-partum
Sex education, in home and schools	**Preconception advice, eg folate supplementation, genetic screening**	**Routine antenatal care**	Anti D programme
MMR immunisation	**Contraception advice**		**Contraception advice, discussion of subsequent pregnancy**

This figure illustrates the range of activity that might improve pregnancy outcome. The bold activities are those where there is a major input from primary care teams

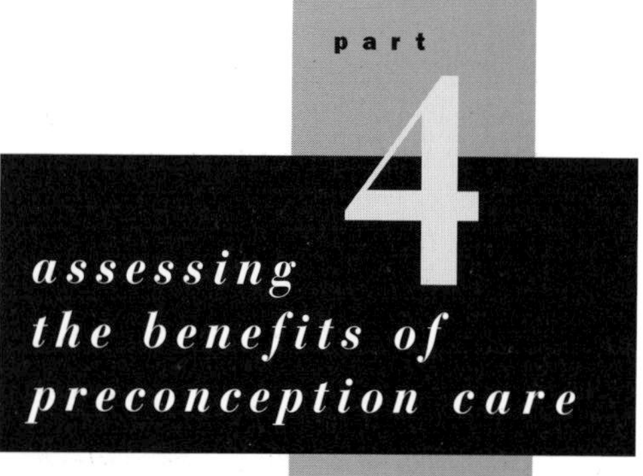

part 4 assessing the benefits of preconception care

Much of the argument in favour of preconception care comes from antenatal care. However present-day antenatal care has been challenged, and Steer has asked whether much of what takes place amounts to ritual behaviour[6].

First, antenatal care consists of a complex system of various actions linked to a number of different outcomes[7]. For instance palpation of the abdomen is undertaken both as a screening examination to assess fetal growth and to check the fetal position (which in turn may be seen to be a crude screen for possible cephalo pelvic disproportion). Second, there is the ethical problem, familiar in other areas, of having to balance potential benefits of a screening programme to those women where treatable conditions are identified at an early stage, with the disadvantages, particularly anxiety and worry, to other women who are incorrectly identified by a positive screening test. The balance between these two factors depends on the positive predictive value of a test. The positive predictive value measures the proportion of women with positive screening tests who truly have the condition. As the prevalence of a condition in the screened population falls the positive predictive value also falls. As the general health of the population improves and the overall risks associated with pregnancy diminish the prevalence of the conditions that are being identified by screening falls, reducing the positive predictive value of the screening tests[8].

Finally there is the 'risk approach paradox', a theoretical problem of assessing the success of screening programmes. The idea is that if a condition is identified at screening and dealt with effectively this represents a problem averted, and this will be recorded as a normal outcome. Effective intervention would appear to diminish the value of a screening test or risk assessment. At the most extreme point, perfectly effective intervention would completely abolish the value of a screening test[9].

There is clear evidence for risks associated with certain habits and medical problems. That does not automatically mean that they constitute a risk both before and after conception. Except in a few specific instances there is very little evidence that supports intervention before, rather than after conception, and very few studies that make direct comparisons between interventions before and after conception. These arguments are illustrated most clearly by evidence on smoking (see below).

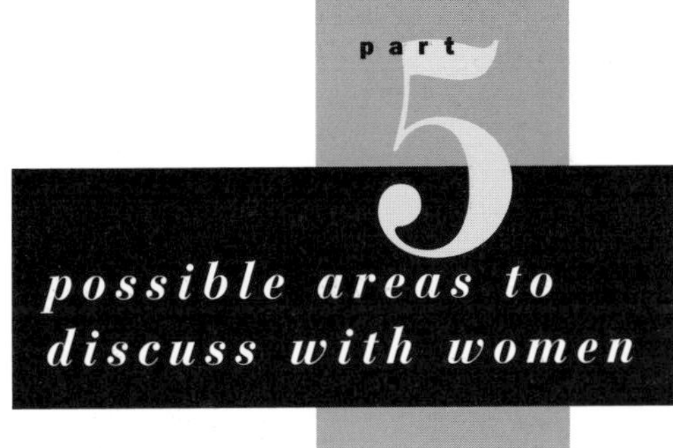

part 5 possible areas to discuss with women

Past obstetric history

The first study to report a preconception service was by Chamberlain, working from a tertiary care centre[10]. Perhaps unsurprisingly, most referrals were to discuss what had happened in the previous pregnancy, with the largest number discussing preterm labour or late miscarriage. Similar figures were reported from a much larger series attending a similar facility in Glasgow[11]. This study admitted that the clinic appeared to have made very little difference to the outcome of subsequent pregnancies in these mothers.

General advice about lifestyle

Smoking is associated with reduced birthweight, increased perinatal mortality rate and a higher rate of preterm delivery[12,13]. Alcohol is also associated with reduced birthweight, and at much higher doses with the fetal alcohol syndrome of growth retardation and characteristic congenital anomalies[14]. Use of cocaine and cannabis have been linked to shorter gestations; cocaine and heroin to intrauterine growth retardation. Opiate abuse causes dependence in newborn infants, and cocaine use has been reported in some studies to be associated with placental abruption[14a]. No particular influence has been ascribed to general dietary intake, except when there is severe famine. Exercise has generally been associated with positive pregnancy outcomes[15].

As was stated above, knowing that certain habits are harmful does not mean that actions taken to discourage them will always do good. There is likely to be benefit in any interventions that are aimed at reducing the rates of congenital anomalies. It may be reasonable to give advice concerning heavy drinking, smoking and opiate abuse at any stage in patients' lives. It is generally believed that women may be better motivated to change habits during pregnancy, although it is hard to find empirical evidence to support this view. The important question from a policy maker's point of view, is whether advice given at this stage confers greater gains than standard advice given during pregnancy. The evidence on smoking is quite clear: giving up at any stage up to four months' gestation puts women and their babies on a par with non-smokers[12,16]. In the only example where a direct comparison has been made, successfully giving up smoking pre-conception is no better for mother and baby than doing so in the first four months of gestation. In contrast one study points out the dangers of lifestyle advice: a group of disadvantaged pregnant women in Glasgow found advice to give up smoking difficult to follow and responded either by discounting the advice or by feeling guilty at their recidivist behaviour[17].

The fetal alcohol syndrome causes major abnormalities and is presumably operating at the stage of conception. Any advice to prevent it would have to be given at or before this time. Such advice would apply only to a small number of very heavy drinkers. If general practitioners had identified such drinkers it is likely that they would encourage the patients to reduce their intake for their own health, in the same way that they would act where opiate abuse is concerned. Women drinking up to 2-3 units of alcohol daily, who comprise the majority of pregnant women, do not seem to be damaging their fetuses when compared with those who don't drink at all[18].

Work

Evidence suggests that women working late in pregnancy have lower rates of preterm delivery and low birthweight babies in both the UK and France[19,20]. However the effect on birthweight disappeared when the data was adjusted for adverse medical or obstetric history. This suggests a 'healthy worker effect', whereby employment selects for healthy individuals.

If in general there is no evidence to suggest women should stop work before or after conception, certain occupations are associated with particular risks. Exposure to anaesthetic gases, most probably nitrous oxide increases the miscarriage rate[21]. Perinatal mortality rate is higher in women working in the chemical and dry cleaning industries, and congenital abnormalities are more frequent among those working in the glass and pottery industries[22]. Working with VDU screens seems to carry no additional risk[23].

There is also the controversial evidence from children born close to the nuclear energy plant at Sellafield that exposure of fathers to radioactivity could be responsible for the increase in leukaemia among the children.

Responding to such information is difficult. Even where clear risks exist it may be very difficult for women and men to take any action to reduce them.

Preventing fetal disease

NEURAL TUBE DEFECTS

The argument for encouraging women to take folic acid supplements before and at the time of conception is well-established. Randomised controlled trials of supplements have demonstrated the benefit of folate supplements in preventing neural tube defects, both in women who have already had one affected child[24] and in first pregnancies[25]. However despite strong recommendations from the Department of the Health, in practice few women are taking folic acid supplements[26] and the debate has now shifted to the arguments for and against fortifying foods with folic acid[27].

INFECTIONS

The practice of establishing the rubella immunity status of women before conception is also well-established. The risk of transmission from mother to fetus is highest in the first trimester. The introduction to the UK of MMR vaccination in the early 1980s should by now be guaranteeing both immunity of the majority of women of childbearing age as well as a substantial population immunity. However checking the rubella status of women at some stage before conception, and offering immunisation to those who are not immune is sensible, and has no discernible contraindications.

Toxoplasma gondii can also be transmitted to fetuses. Among women who seroconvert in the course of their pregnancies only a minority of fetuses are infected, and fewer than half of them develop the cerebral complications. The screening programme in France is one that occurs during pregnancy (not before or around conception) and consists of repeated serological tests for toxoplasma infection. The argument against screening in the UK is that infection is less common, but also that treatment for infections is less than completely effective at eradicating the infection[28]. For non-immune women who are concerned, the standard advice would be to avoid any contact with cat faeces, although the value of such advice is not established. Similarly Listeria monocytogenes is a known source of congenital infection and can cause second trimester miscarriage[29]. It may be found in unpasteurised milk, soft cheeses, and pates. While it would appear sensible to advise women to avoid such foods, it is not clear that such advice can in practice achieve anything other than generating more anxiety.

GENETIC DISORDERS

Advising and testing for genetic disorders is likely to become an increasingly important part of general practice in the future, and will generate its own need for preconception advice. Carrier screening can already be offered for cystic fibrosis, beta thalassaemia, sickle cell disease, and Tay-Sachs disease. Screening for fragile X syndrome has been recommended and is currently under discussion. There is scope for testing for genes associated with increased risk of diabetes, ischaemic heart disease and particular cancersThe human gene project will surely uncover further possibilities on a large scale. Testing for the four commonest cystic fibrosis genes was broadly acceptable to women attending antenatal clinics in primary care, with a small and transient increase in anxiety when awaiting the result[30]. In this study testing was offered either to women, with partners screened only if the women were positive, or to couples together. Unfortunately it is unclear whether the test was acceptable to men and women equally. Uptake rates were low when offered to a general practice population, where the women were not pregnant[31].

Testing means dealing with positive tests. When women who had been tested for cystic fibrosis mutations were asked why they had accepted the test, and what they would have done if it had been positive, there was a clear statement that they accepted any test offered in pregnancy, and that only a minority had worked out exactly how they would respond to a positive test[32]. Some tests are for diseases such as sickle cell disease which may be mild in their effects, or such as cystic fibrosis where the treatment is improving to the point where some sufferers may lead completely normal lives. Under such circumstances not all parents will choose to terminate affected pregnancies.

The future for genetic screening is unpredictable. At present there is not large scale support for routine carrier screening of everybody, perhaps at school leaving age, but it is possible to imagine public perception changing very rapidly as there is more understanding of the new genetics.[33] However it is likely that increasing numbers of men and women will wish to discuss their personal family histories of disease to assess the likelihood of a genetic factor and the possibility to screen for it. Primary care teams need to know how to take and record family history to assess the risk of genetic disease, to be informed about facilities available locally for testing, and to be able to help their patients make decisions and deal with the 'genetic guilt' when tests reveal a genetic abnormality.

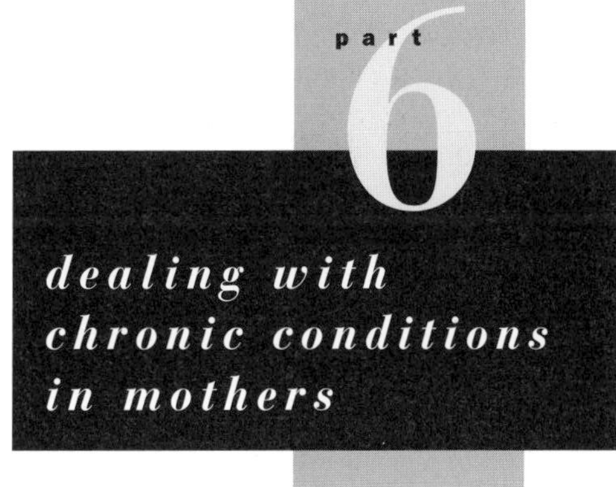

The important aspects to consider are:

- the effect on the health of the mother
- the possibility of genetic inheritance of a disease or defect
- the possibility of the pregnancy causing a deterioration in the condition in question
- the possibility of the disease or its treatment causing some other congenital problem

In the experience of a prepregnancy clinic in Glasgow, women with chronic disease formed the only group where outcome in the subsequent pregnancy was improved by attendance at the clinic[11].

Pregnancy in diabetic women carries well-known complications to the fetuses: high rates of late intrauterine death, and large babies with the potential for difficult labour. Congenital malformations are also more common in the babies of diabetic women, and there is a body of evidence that good glycaemic control is associated with lower rates of complications. There is, then, a clear argument in favour of giving advice and help for closer monitoring of blood sugar levels before and around the time of conception. There is controversy whether advice is best provided in dedicated pre-pregnancy clinics. One review suggested that such clinics merely separated diabetic women into well-motivated attenders with good control and non-attenders with poor control[34].

The position of women with other chronic diseases is less clear. There are very few conditions, for instance Eisenmenger's syndrome and pulmonary hypertension, where pregnancy is associated with high maternal mortality.

The commonest problem, of possible teratogenic effects of drugs being taken to control a particular condition, is rarely simple. It requires a balance to be struck between the need to maintain control of the condition, and the risk, usually small, of teratogenesis. In some cases, for instance in women with epilepsy or hypertension, there is sufficient knowledge to make it worth changing women from drugs with known teratogenic effects to others[35].

Primary care teams should make sure that all women with such conditions are aware, before they become pregnant, that there may be implications for pregnancy. Women with diabetes can be given clear advice. For others it is likely to be less clear, but they are entitled to the best information to enable them to make their own choices.

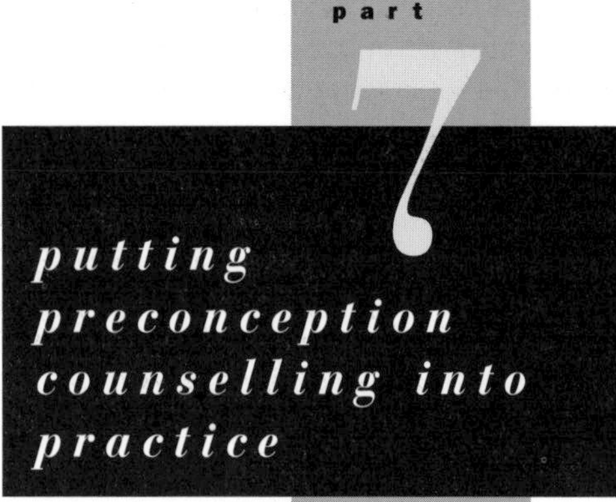

part 7 putting preconception counselling into practice

The evidence, as summarised above, might justify setting up some form of preconception service. However there has been a retreat from the position of seeing all prevention as an unqualified blessing.

Concerns have been raised both about the extent of benefits to be gained, and about the possible consequences, both of raising unnecessary anxiety among the healthy and of giving false reassurance to those who are less healthy. In addition services that have been offered tend to be used more by those who need them less – the so called worried well. This has been coupled with an awareness, from ethical considerations, that when professionals offer to give advice or help in areas that are not previously considered by patients to be matters of concern, there is a particular obligation to be confident of doing more good than harm. However we genuinely don't know if we would be doing harm, and it is legitimate to question the wisdom of any moves that may tend to medicalise the act of conception.

Limits to what can be achieved

Even when contraception is widely available, many live and welcomed babies begin as unintended pregnancies. The most recent studies report rates between 27 per cent and 65 per cent[36,37]. The reasons may be more subtle than simple contraceptive errors[38].

Therefore any move to offer advice to women planning to conceive is likely to be severely limited in terms of the benefits to be achieved. If an intervention is to be offered to all women before conception, then leaving it up to them to come asking for the advice as part of a planned pregnancy will result in limited coverage. For many of those who attended such a service, no specific intervention would be indicated, although one study put the figure as high as 38 per cent of women potentially benefiting from preconception counselling[39].

The generalists' approach

The obvious answer is to identify other opportunities to pass on such advice. AS GPs in the UK we have the enormous advantage of seeing a large proportion of our patients for other purposes. In particular we see many women of childbearing age for contraceptive advice. Even this is unlikely to represent a perfect solution. The extent to which doctors feel able to discuss preparation for conception at a consultation whose primary purpose is to discuss contraception will depend on both doctors and patients. Quite apart from ignoring fundamental precepts of adult education, offering information to women at precisely the time that it is of no use to them may lead to confusion.

In the light of these difficulties, and the limited range of interventions that can be advocated wholeheartedly, it would be prudent to adopt a restrained view of preconception advice. This excludes anything to imply that women should be coming to discuss conception with professionals, or that they would be acting more responsibly if they did so. What is needed is an approach both broader in its overall approach in some areas and better targeted in others. We do not need to feel defensive or defeatist about the limited gains to be achieved by a specific service provided we identify a much wider range of services that can make a contribution, however indirect, to maternal and child health, much of which is already taking place. A possible list of interventions is given opposite.

- **Education of any kind, in any setting, designed to increase men and women's understanding of sexual health. This would comprise information about conception and contraception, but would also include information about smoking and diet**

- **Contraceptive services that enable men and women to plan their conceptions. This would include provision of services for therapeutic abortions**

- **Services offered at a level of general practice, to all patients, that may have a bearing on maternal and child health. Such services would include provision of rubella immunisation programmes, practice policies on encouraging the stopping of smoking, etc**

- **Making use of other opportunities such as consultations for contraception, to offer advice about conception, provided it is not found to be intrusive by the patients**

- **Any policies to support peri-conceptual folic acid supplementation**

- **Offering explicitly to discuss conception with any women planning a pregnancy, should they request it**

- **Encouraging nulliparous young women with identified chronic disease, or women who might be carriers for genetic disease, to consider the specific problems of pregnancy, and to offer advice appropriate for that condition**

Consulting with women who request preconception advice

For those who request it the prime duty must be, as always, not to harm. Even given a minimalist approach it is possible to pass on a lot of advice that may convey a picture of pregnancy as being a highly risky enterprise. A possible checklist is suggested below:

- What is the couple's prime concern (if any)?
- Are there any specific risks associated with their personal and family histories (family history of genetically transmitted disease, chronic illness or drug ingestion in the woman, work history of man and woman)?
- Is there any aspect of the previous obstetric history that may be causing concern?
- Does the woman know that she is immune to rubella?
- Does she keep a record of her periods, and does she know when is the time she is most likely to conceive?
- Discuss aspects of smoking, drinking alcohol, exercise, diet (including if appropriate advice to avoid listeria infection)
- Advise folate supplementation

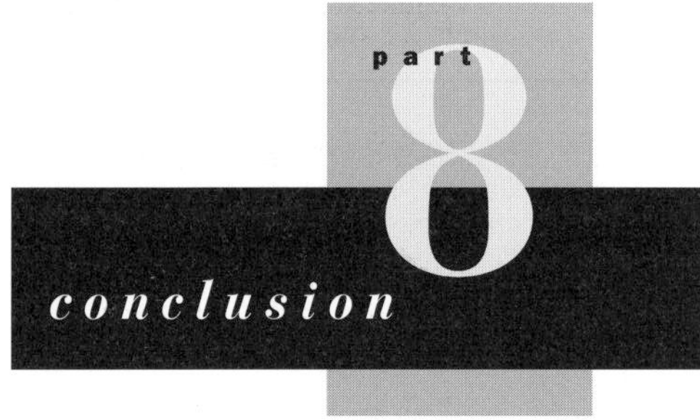

The literature reveals only a limited number of areas where there is clear and convincing evidence of the benefit of advice or intervention specifically given preconception: rubella immunisation, folic acid supplementation, care given to women with chronic disease, specifically diabetes mellitus, and the programme to prevent rhesus sensitisation. On the other hand there is continuing evidence that many pregnancies are unplanned and there will always be limited scope for any programme of preconception care reaching anything approaching the majority of women before or at the time of conception. Recent experience with 'health promotion' should discourage both GPs and the Department of Health from setting out on enterprises where there is a risk of a substantial mismatch between the effort required and the likely health gains. Yet the idea of preconception care continues to exercise a grip on medicine's desire to create a perfect world. Searching Medline revealed a substantial increase in the number of references indexed under 'preconception' over the last few years (not all of which were concerned with research into folic acid supplementation). General practice does not need to repeat this mistake: accepting the broader view of what constitutes preconception care implies that we can encourage and claim credit for a wide range of activities that offer wide-ranging, if modest benefits to all the women in our care.

Evidence suggests that dedicated preconception clinics would offer a poor return for the effort that would be required in setting them up and running them. Adopting a much broader approach towards a definition of preconception care can enable general practitioners to recognise a major contribution that many of them will already be making to the health of pregnant women.

part 10 references

1 'Cerebral palsy, intrapartum care, and a shot in the foot', Anonymous, ***Lancet, 2,*** 1989, 1251-52

2 ***Changing childbirth,*** Expert Maternity Group, HMSO, 1993

3 'Screening for carriers of cystic fibrosis: screening before pregnancy is needed' Raeburn JA, Expert Maternity Group, ***British Medical Journal, 309,*** 1994, 1428-29

4 'Screening for carriers of cystic fibrosis. Psychological consequences are unclear', Marteau T, ***British Medical Journal, 309,*** 1994, 1429-30

5 'Short, Black, Baird, Himsworth, and social class and differences in fetal and neonatal mortality rates', Chalmers I, ***British Medical Journal, 291,*** 1985, 231-33 (N)

6 'Rituals in antenatal care - do we need them?', Steer P, ***British Medical Journal, 307,*** 1993, 697-98

7 ***Screening and surveillance in general practice*** Hart CR and Burke P (eds), 'Antenatal and postnatal care', Jewell D, Churchill Livingstone, 1992, 103-20

8 ***Effectiveness and satisfaction in antenatal care,*** Enkin M and Chalmers I (eds), 'Screening and diagnostic tests in antenatal care', Grant A and Mohide P, Heinemann Medical Books, 1982, 22-59,

9 ***Advances in Perinatal Medicine. v.*** 4, Milunsky A, Friedman E and Gluck L (eds), 'Assessing risk assessment', 235-66, Peters T and Golding J, Plenum Medical Book Company, New York, 1985

10 'The prepregnancy clinic', Chamberlain G, ***British Medical Journal, 281,*** 1980, 29-30

11 'Prepregnancy counselling: experience from 1,075 cases', Cox M, Whittle MJ and Byrne A, et al, ***British Journal of Obstetrics & Gynaecology, 99,*** 1992, 873-76

12 'Cigarette smoking in pregnancy: its influence on birth weight and perinatal mortality', Butler NR, Goldstein H and Ross EM, ***British Medical Journal, 2,*** 1972, 127-30

13 'Factors associated with spontaneous pre-term birth' Fedrick J and Anderson BM, ***British Journal of Obstetrics & Gynaecology, 83,*** 1976, 342-50

14 Recognition of the fetal alchohol syndrome in early infancy, Jones KL and Smith DW, ***Lancet, 2,*** 1973, 999-1001

14a 'Women and substance abuse', Stein MD and Cyr MG, ***Medical Clinics of North America, 81,*** 1997, 979-98

15 'Maternal and fetal responses to a maternal aerobic exercise program', Collings CA, Curet LB and Mullin JP, ***American Journal of Obstetrics & Gynecology, 145,*** 1983, 702-7

16 'Smoking in pregnancy: effects of stopping at different stages' MacArthur C and Knox EG, ***British Journal of Obstetrics & Gynaecology 1988, 95,*** 551-55

17 'Smoking in pregnancy: the attitudes of expectant mothers', Graham H ***Social Science and Medicine, 10,*** 1976, 399-405

18 'Is moderate drinking associated with an increased risk for malformation?', Mills JL and Graubard BI, ***Pediatrics, 80,*** 1987, 309-14

19 'Pregnant women at work', Saurel MJ and Kaminski M, ***Lancet, 1,*** 1983, 475

20 'Employment in pregnancy: prevalence, maternal characteristics, perinatal outcome', Murphy JF , Dauncey M and Newcombe R, et al, ***Lancet, 1,*** 1984, 1163-66

21 'Occupational hazards of anaesthesia', Vessey MP and Nunn JF, ***British Medical Journal, 281,*** 1980, 696-98

22 ***Pregnant women at work: short- and long-term associations,*** Chamberlain G, Peters TJ and Adelstein P, et al (eds), 'The effects of work in pregnancy', Butler NR, Royal Society of Medicine, 1984,87-104

23 'Video display terminals and pregnancy. A review', Blackwell R and Chang A, ***British Journal of Obstetrics & Gynaecology, 95,*** 1988, 446-53

24 'Prevention of neural tube defects: results of the Medical Research Council Vitamin Study', MRC Vitamin Study Research Group, ***Lancet, 338,*** 1991, 131-37

25 'Prevention of the first occurrence of neural-tube defects by periconceptional vitamin supplementation', Czeizel AE and Dudas I, ***New England Journal of Medicine, 327,*** 1992, 1832-5

26 'Minimal compliance with the Department of Health recommendation for routine folate prophylaxis to prevent neural tube defects', Clark NAC and Fisk NM, ***British Journal of Obstetrics & Gynaecology, 101,*** 1994, 709-10

27 'Folic acid and the prevention of neural tube defects', Wald NJ and Bower C, ***British Medical Journal, 310,*** 1995, 1019-20

28 'Toxoplasmosis in pregnancy and its transmission to the fetus', Desmonts G and Couvreur J, ***Bulletin of the New York Academy of Medicine, 50,*** 1947, 146-59

29 'Listeria', Spencer JAD, ***British Medical Journal, 295,*** 1987, 349

29a 'Screening for fragile X is cost effective and accurate', ***British Medical Journal, 315,*** 1997, 208

30 'Cystic fibrosis carrier testing in early pregnancy by general practitioners', Harris H, Scotcher D and Hartley N, et al, ***British Medical Journal, 306,*** 1993, 1580-83

31 'Uptake of cystic fibrosis testing in primary care: supply push or demand pull?', Bekker H, Modell M and Denniss G, et al, ***British Medical Journal, 306,*** 1993, 1584-86

32 'Pilot study of the acceptability of cysic fibrosis carrier testing during routine antenatal consultations in general practice', Harris H, Scotcher D and Hartley N, et al, ***British Journal of General Practice, 46,*** 1996, 225-7

33 'Screening for cystic fibrosis in primary care', Burn J ***British Medical Journal, 306,*** 1993, 1558-59

34 Are diabetic pre-pregnancy clinics worth while?, Gregory R and Tattersall RB, ***Lancet, 340,*** 1992, 656-8

35 'Preconceptional counseling and intervention', Kuller JA and Laifer SA, ***Archives of internal Medicine, 154,*** 1994, 2273-80

36 'Lessons from an audit of unplanned pregnancies', Metson D, ***British Medical Journal, 297,*** 1988, 904-6

37 Factors related to planned and unplanned pregnancies, Rosenfeld JA and Everett KD, ***Journal of Family Practice, 43,*** 1996,161-66

38 ***Taking chances: abortion and the decision not to contracept***, Luker K, Berkley, Los Angeles, 1975

39 'Pregnancy planning and pre-conception counselling', Adams MM et al The PRAMS Working Group, ***Journal of Obstetrics & Gynecology, 82,*** 1993, 955-59

Acknowledgements

I would like to thank Catriona Erskine for her valuable contribution to this chapter.

David Jewell

Catherine Paterson

chapter eight

unplanned pregnancy

part

I

introduction

Becoming pregnant and having a child can be one of life's greatest experiences, but much of the joy is based on it being a wanted child. Control of fertility is central to contentment and prosperity. People need to be able to plan their lives, and almost without exception they see having a child as an opportunity to give that child a good life. For a woman, being able to become pregnant may be central to her life. Even those who never see themselves wanting children, or see having children as an activity for the future, treasure the ability to choose.

part

2

diagnosis of pregnancy

It is important for women to have easy access to pregnancy testing. There is significant stress associated with a late period and a woman may present to her GP for a pregnancy test, or she may already know that she is pregnant. It is important that the first health professional to have contact does not make any assumptions about the pregnancy. A woman may be clearly delighted or just shocked. In either case she may need time to think about the pregnancy, and it will often be appropriate for her to spend some time with her partner, friends or family before making any definitive plans. An unplanned pregnancy may not be unwanted – at least 33 per cent of continuing pregnancies are unplanned but nevertheless happy events. Alternatively some planned pregnancies may become unwanted. This most commonly occurs when a relationship breaks down, or it may follow prenatal diagnosis of a fetal anomaly.

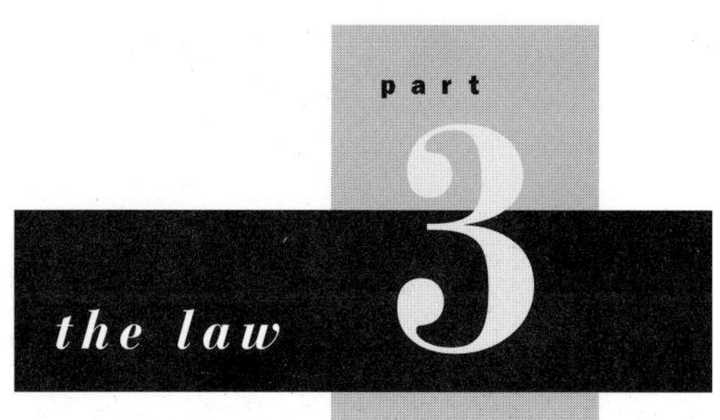

part 3 the law

The Abortion Act as amended in 1991, demands that two doctors certify in good faith that one or more of the following grounds are met:

a the continuation of the pregnancy would involve risk to the life of the pregnant woman greater than if the pregnancy were terminated

b the termination is necessary to prevent grave permanent injury to the physical or mental health of the pregnant woman

c the pregnancy has not exceeded its 24th week and that the continuance of the pregnancy would involve risk, greater than if the pregnancy were terminated, of injury to the physical or mental health of the pregnant woman

d the pregnancy has not exceeded its 24th week and that the continuance of the pregnancy would involve risk, greater than if the pregnancy were terminated, of injury to the physical or mental health of any existing child(ren) of the family of the pregnant woman

e there is substantial risk that if the child were born it would suffer from such physical or mental abnormalities as to be seriously handicapped.

In practice these often divide into 'social' grounds (clauses c and d) and medical grounds (clauses a, b and e). Clause e is mainly used in association with antenatal services offering prenatal screening and diagnoses, and women undergoing termination of a 'wanted' pregnancy have special needs. The stillbirth and neonatal death society (SANDS) publishes guidelines for professionals which have information about funerals, grieving and the need for genetic counselling. SATFA (Support after Termination for Fetal Abnormality) also offers guidance and support (see *Useful organisations*, page 195).

The law can be interpreted liberally but does not permit abortion on request. A doctor needs to identify factors threatening mental health. However most women who wish to have an abortion should be able to find two doctors willing to support her request. In practice the limiting factor is usually local NHS provision. A woman who is able to fund her abortion and is free to travel to an independent abortion clinic should be able to get an abortion providing that she does not have a medical condition that makes abortion in a 'stand alone' clinic contraindicated.

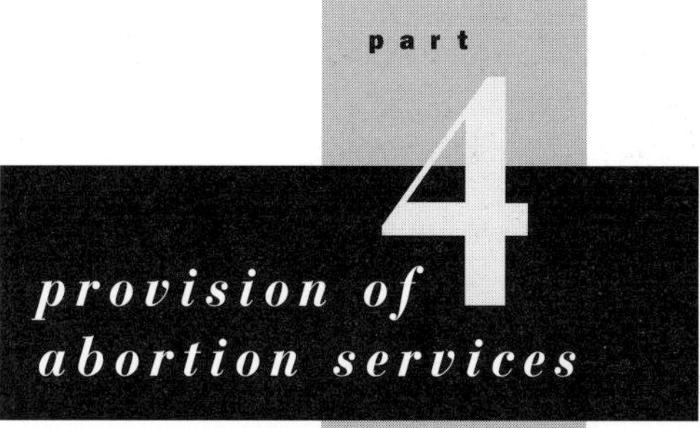

part 4 provision of abortion services

NHS services may be purchased by the health authority or GP fundholders, and provided by an NHS hospital or specialist providers, such as the British Pregnancy Advisory Service or Marie Stopes (non profit-making organisations). A woman may also pay for her own abortion at a specialised clinic or via a private gynaecologist.

The proportion of abortions paid for by the NHS varies widely in different parts of the country, from less than 30 per cent to over 97 per cent[1]. Provision is improving as the decision to provide abortion services is now taken by purchasing health authorities rather than by individual hospitals. Where hospitals are unable or unwilling to provide abortions, the service may be purchased from specialist providers.

The ease of getting a self-funded abortion may depend on the geographical proximity of independent abortion clinics for women who choose, or are forced, to pay for their abortion.

Where there is limited NHS provision the health authority may introduce criteria such as age, gestation, receipt of supplementary benefit, unemployment, refugee status or more than a certain number of children, that need to be fulfilled before a woman is able to have an abortion on the NHS. It is important to be aware that it may be possible for a GP to arrange for the purchasing authority to pay for an abortion for a woman who is unable to get one through routine channels but whom the GP feels has special needs. Women who have to 'bargain' for a NHS abortion are often unable to be honest about their true feelings or to resolve any personal ambivalence before their termination of pregnancy.

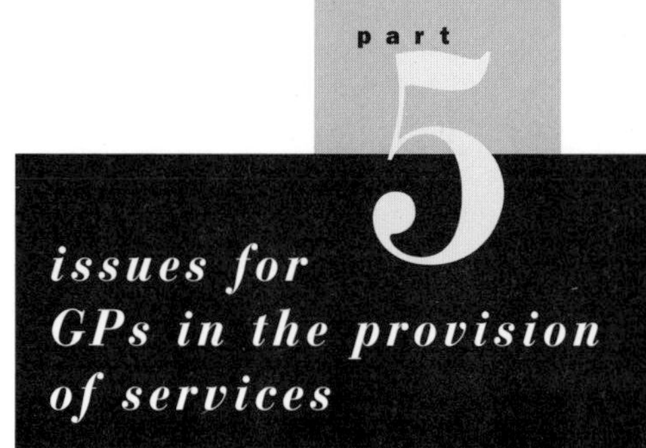

part 5 issues for GPs in the provision of services

It is important that a practice should have up-to-date information on local provision. This includes the percentage provided by the health authority, how to access the service, the average waiting times for assessment and abortion, any gestation or 'social' restrictions, the methods used and whether contraceptive advice and/or supplies are provided. The price and availability of self-funded abortions should also be available.

It is beneficial for a woman to be seen 1-2 weeks after her abortion to confirm that she is well, to answer queries about the abortion and to ensure that she is happy with her method of contraception. Some services may offer a follow-up visit, but in most cases the woman will return to the referring doctor and this visit should be encouraged.

There should be a strategy for GPs unable to support abortion requests and an understanding within the practice that personal freedom of choice is not only important for doctors, but also for women who are overwhelmingly the ones affected by an unwanted child. There is a moral and professional responsibility to direct a woman to a doctor who can give unbiased information, and support for abortion if requested.

The practice should know the procedure for getting an abortion for a woman where she would be unable to go through routine channels. For example where the waiting time puts the pregnancy over the gestation limit, a medical condition which means that she is unable to have an abortion under an agency contract, or where she may not fulfil health authority criteria but still be unable to support a child. Often women within these categories, particularly those who present late, are the ones most in need of an abortion. Arranging an abortion under these circumstances may involve discussion with the local provider, or referral to an alternative one.

The practice policy in relation to abortion and confidentiality, particularly for women under 16, should be stated in the practice leaflet. The position in relation to under 16s is clearly discussed in a booklet published by the Brook Advisory Centres[1a].

Health visitors or practice nurses may be the first to be approached, particularly if they do pregnancy testing, and should be able to give information and support to a woman with an unplanned pregnancy. Even when a woman has a good relationship with her GP she may not feel able to discuss her need for an abortion with him/her and should be able to get a direct referral for an abortion. This may be via the family planning or genitourinary medicine clinic.

A woman who has her request for abortion sympathetically and effectively handled is much more likely to return for further advice relating to sexual health.

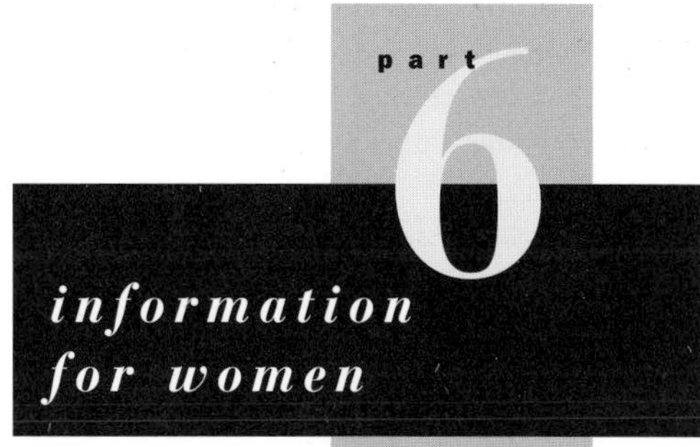

part 6 *information for women*

It is important to be able to discuss the alternatives to abortion if requested. This might include social support, temporary fostering or adoption and requre referral to social services for further information.

The information that women seek is often included in the following questions:

- Will I be able to become pregnant in the future?
- How long will I have to wait for the abortion?
- Will it hurt?
- How long does the operation take?
- What happens?
- Will anybody else find out about the abortion?
- How big is the fetus?
- Will it feel pain?
- What happens to the fetal tissue after the abortion?
- What might go wrong?

Most of these are answered in the text. Many women with an unplanned pregnancy feel protective towards the fetus, especially as pregnancy advances, and may be concerned about fetal issues such as the size of the fetus, the ability of the fetus to feel pain and the disposal of fetal matter. All questions should be answered accurately – if a woman does not want to know she will not ask. Although a fetus may respond to a noxious stimulus there is no scientific evidence of sentient behaviour before 26 weeks' gestation[2]. Women may be further reassured that if an abortion is performed under general anaesthesia both the woman and her fetus will be anaesthetised. Fetal tissue is disposed of by incineration. In some units this may be a dedicated incinerater, in others one dedicated to human tissue. Intact fetuses may be cremated and within our Trust this is performed with a non denominational service on a monthly basis.

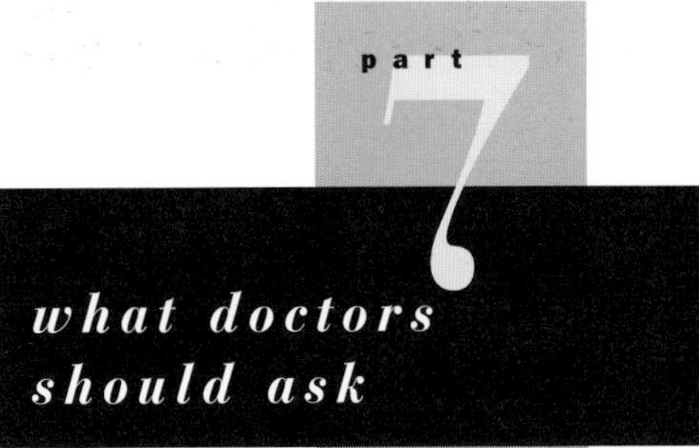

part 7 what doctors should ask

A doctor should ask why the woman wants an abortion. Occasionally women have unfounded anxieties about the outcome of a particular pregnancy. For example a woman with myxoedema diagnosed after her first pregnancy stopped her thyroxine immediately she realised that she was pregnant. She was concerned that the drug would have damaged the fetus and was requesting an abortion. When it was explained that the drug would not harm the fetus, and that it was important to have adequate levels of thyroxine she restarted her medication and continued with her unplanned but wanted pregnancy.

The doctor should ask if the woman is certain that she wants an abortion, and if not that she knows about the alternatives. S/he should ask whether the decision has been discussed with the woman's partner /parents/friends, and what effect she thinks that the pregnancy and/or abortion will have on her relationship with them. It may be helpful to discuss future fertility plans, these may influence her final decision.

Referral for abortion should contain a brief outline of the reasons for requesting abortion, parity, the last menstrual period and clinical gestation (particularly if there is a discrepancy), any medical problems and medication and any decision about contraception (if discussed). Most units ask the referring doctor to enclose a signed HSA1 (blue) form.

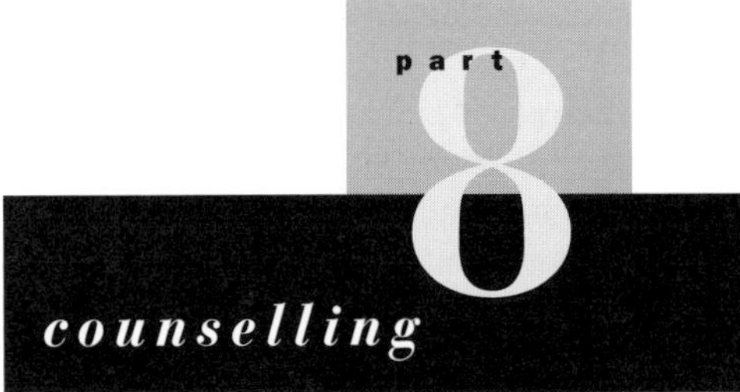

part 8 counselling

Not all women require formal counselling but all need an opportunity to talk through their decision and get accurate information about abortion and the alternatives. The GP may be the first to see a woman after the pregnancy has been diagnosed and should be able provide this.

Much counselling that is required is centred around relationships rather than the actual abortion and women who do not have a good personal support system (reduced support may be related to the need for confidentiality, particularly in groups where unmarried sexual relationships and/or abortion is not allowed) need an unbiased person with whom to talk things through. While abortion is often seen as the only realistic practical solution to the pregnancy it is important that a woman is able to discuss fears and misgivings, without feeling that airing these will jeopardise her chance of getting an abortion.

Many women worry more about other people's reaction to their abortion rather their own and it is helpful if someone can give them the support required to make the decision most appropriate for and acceptable to themselves. In the end it is the woman who most has to live with the outcome of her decision.

It is important that a woman understands that it must be her own decision. It is not uncommon for women, especially young ones, to ask permission to have an abortion: 'Do you think I should have the baby, or have an abortion?' It is inevitable that any decision will be influenced by the people around her – they are the part of the fabric of her life. Having a baby when partner and parents are delighted and able to offer both financial and emotional support is very different to financially supporting a child when there is an aura of disapproval and lack of emotional support. Only the woman herself can make the choice and she should be given the freedom to do so, but with freedom comes the need to take responsibility for the action and to understand that, like any decision, there is a possibility that it is the wrong one. Women who really want the child or feel unable to have an abortion will usually find a solution to the practical problems and should be offered support.

There may be language and cultural barriers when discussing abortion. A close family member may not be a suitable independent interpreter and where possible a professional interpreter or advocate who is familiar with the woman's language and culture should be present for discussions. This facility may be available at the clinic.

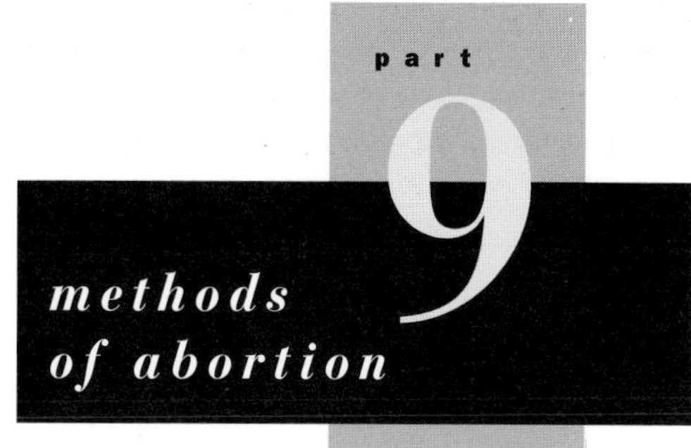

Methods of abortion depend on gestation, the facilities available, and, where choice is available, the wishes of the woman[3,4].

Early medical abortion (up to 9 weeks' gestation)

Mifepristone (RU486) is an orally active progesterone antagonist[5], currently licensed for the termination of pregnancies at less than 63 days' gestation, at a dose of 600mg (3 tablets) followed by 1mg vaginal gemeprost 36-48 hours later. Mifepristone appears to be a very safe drug with few side effects and most contraindications to medical abortions relate to the concomitant use of a prostaglandin.

There have been many studies looking at the dose of mifepristone and the WHO demonstrated that a single dose of 200mg was as effective as 600mg[6]. The current recommended dose of prostaglandin has also been challenged[7], and Penny et al[8] demonstrated that 800mcg of the orally active prostaglandin analogue given vaginally was 95 per cent effective at less than 49 days' gestation and 93 per cent effective between 49 and 63 days. Because of its low cost and reduced prostaglandin side effects this alternative (unlicensed) regime may be used in some units.

The woman will be asked to attend the unit providing the abortion to take the mifepristone 2 days before admission as a day case for the prostaglandin and actual abortion. She should be told that in the interim she can continue normal activities. About 40 per cent will have some vaginal bleeding and between 1 and 3 per cent may abort prior to admission. This is not usually alarming and the woman should be given a 24 hour contact number for advice in case she has any concerns.

Thirty-six to 48 hours later the woman will be admitted to the unit providing the abortion for prostaglandin administration. Following this the onset of bleeding and uterine contractions is variable. All women will be asked to use a commode so that the products of conception can be seen as soon as they are passed. Seventy per cent will abort within 4 hours. If the passage of products is not confirmed within 8 hours the woman may scanned or be allowed to go home to return for a scan a few days later. The continuing pregnancy rate is about 1 per cent and surgical evacuation for partial retained products of conception may be required in about 4 per cent, although the majority of women with prolonged vaginal loss will respond to conservative management.

Suction termination of pregnancy (6-13 weeks' gestation)

This is the most common method of abortion for the 90 per cent that are performed in the first trimester. It is normally a day case procedure and may be performed under local or general anaesthetic and takes about 10 minutes. In the UK most procedures are performed under general anaesthesia. It is a safe procedure but women should be aware of the small risks or anaesthesia, surgical complications (uterine perforation or cervical damage) pelvic infection, retained products of conception requiring re-evacuation and, particularly at very early gestations, the very small risk of an ongoing pregnancy. These risks can be minimised by careful preoperative assessment, cervical preparation[9], an experienced surgeon, and either preoperative screening for vaginal infections or the use of prophylactic antibiotics[10]. Most women can return to normal activities the next day.

Dilatation and evacuation (13-20 weeks' gestation)

The provision of dilatation and evacuation (D&E) varies between units. Some will only provide surgical termination of pregnancy in the first trimester and those who do provide D&E may only do so to 14,16 or 18 weeks. The procedure is generally performed under general anaesthesia following cervical preparation with either prostaglandins or hygroscopic cervical dilators (Dilapan or laminaria). It involves wider cervical dilatation and removal of the products of conception piecemeal. The risks are similar to abortion in the first trimester but surgical complications may require more major surgery and/or blood transfusion.

A few units provide surgical termination to 23 weeks' gestation by using a 2 stage procedure. At the first the umbilical cord is divided to cause fetal death and hygroscopic dilators are placed in the cervix. At the second, 24 hours later, the pregnancy is evacuated.

Late medical termination of pregnancy (13-23 weeks' gestation)

This procedure requires admission to hospital, usually overnight. Labour is induced using prostaglandins and the fetus and placenta are delivered whole. An anaesthetic is not required unless the placenta is retained and it can be a painful and distressing procedure for a woman, particularly if she is nulliparous. The woman will normally be offered Entonox and/or parenteral analgesia during the later stages of the abortion. Mifepristone may be given 48 hours prior to admission for the abortion and significantly reduces the induction to abortion period and it is unusual for the procedure to exceed 24 hours, the majority abort within 12 hours. The prostaglandin may be given vaginally or intra-amniotically.

If the pregnancy is more than 20 weeks' gestation it is important to ensure that there are no signs of life at abortion and this is usually achieved either by giving intrauterine urea, or giving a fetal intracardiac injection of potassium chloride under ultrasound guidance.

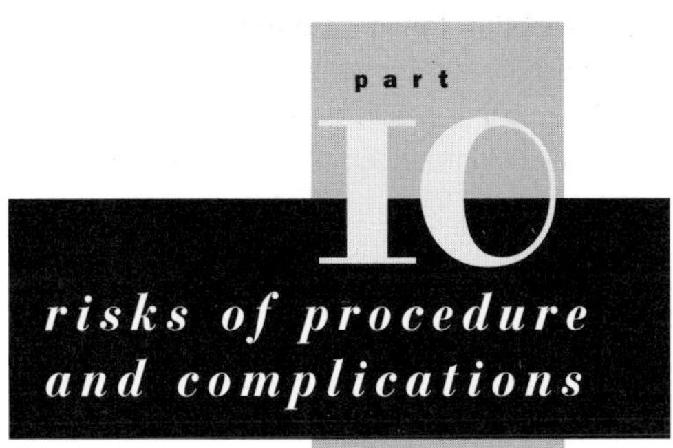

part 10 risks of procedure and complications

Termination of pregnancy is a very safe procedure with a low complication rate, but no procedure can be guaranteed free from risk[11].

Complications can be considered in three groups: immediate, short term and long term.

Immediate

Every anaesthetic carries a small risk, which is influenced by the health of the woman. The majority are young and fit, but some will have medical conditions which have influenced their decision to have an abortion. In these the risk may be significant but needs to be balanced against the risks of carrying a pregnancy to term.

The surgical risk is small but increases with gestation. All women should be made aware of the risk of cervical damage or uterine perforation requiring laparoscopy or laparotomy. In most cases, If promptly diagnosed and managed, it is unlikely that such trauma will affect future reproductive performance. Perforation of the uterus is unusual occurring in about 1 in 500 cases.

Particularly in late abortion, or where there is a surgical complication, there is a small risk of bleeding requiring blood transfusion. If there is serious trauma or bleeding a hysterectomy may be required and death associated with induced abortion occurs in 0.6/1,000,000 women.

Short-term complications

These are usually related to retained products of conception and/or pelvic infection. Pelvic infection can be reduced by prophylactic antibiotics but all women should be aware of the risk of requiring a second procedure to evacuate retained products of conception. The risk may be as high as 1:30.

Irregular bleeding is normal for up to 10 days following an abortion and although abortion is not a painful procedure a woman may get some uterine cramping after the operation which is usually relieved by non steroidal anti inflammatory drugs. However it is important that she reports persistent pain, bleeding or any pyrexia to a doctor.

There is a small risk of ongoing pregnancy, particularly when surgical abortion is performed at less than 6 weeks' gestation, or if there is a double uterus. It is also possible to overlook an ectopic pregnancy and any symptoms of pregnancy, particularly persisting nausea or breast tenderness should be investigated. It is important to remember that even following a successful abortion the pregnancy test may remain positive for up to 3 weeks and a pelvic ultrasound scan and quantitative beta human chorionic gonadotrophin measurements may be required to clarify the situation[12].

Long-term complications

An uncomplicated abortion does not appear to have any effect on future reproductive performance.

Women may feel sad that they had an unplanned pregnancy that they felt unable to continue but even under these circumstances are relieved that they have been able to have an abortion. Regret may be based on a further change in circumstances – life is a dynamic process a woman can only make decisions for today based on the position today and her current perception of the immediate and far future. However the future is always unknown. Mental state after abortion closely correlates to mental state prior to unplanned pregnancy. It is unlikely the abortion per se leads to psychiatric morbidity (on the contrary abortion is usually accompanied by a sense of relief) but the events surrounding unplanned pregnancy, which may often be associated with the break-up of a previously untested but apparently good relationship, may induce stress[13,14].

There is a small risk of tubal damage which may lead to infertility in woman who have unrecognised or untreated pelvic infection. Failure to conceive may not be related to the abortion. For example fertility declines with age and women should be made aware of this prior to the abortion (see also Chapter 6, Table 3 page 106).

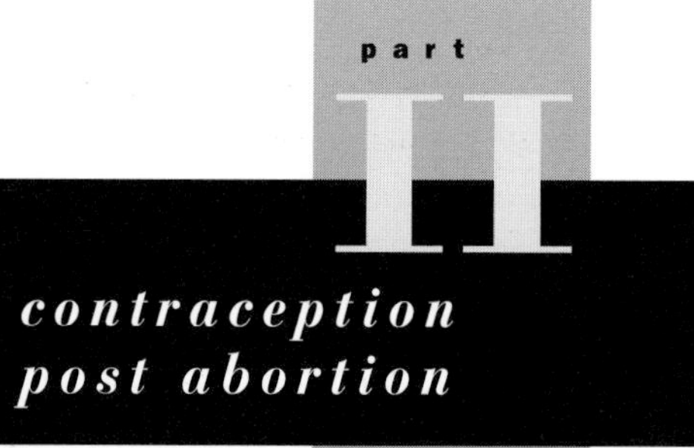

part II contraception post abortion

Some women with an unintended pregnancy are very concerned about contraception and may see this as a priority, while others are so concerned about the pregnancy that they find it difficult to think about contraception. While it is probably not the best time to make any long term decisions about contraception, such as contraceptive implants or sterilisation, it is important to have a short term plan. Women are very vulnerable after an abortion, and, especially when relationships are unstable, may be at risk of unplanned sexual intercourse.

The choice of a contraceptive method will be influenced by a woman's previous experiences, and her background level of knowledge. It is important to understand why contraception failed or was not used. A satisfactory method may have been stopped because of a problem that can easily resolved, or unfounded fears about the risks or long term effects of a given method. A consultation relating to an unplanned pregnancy may be a good time to give information, and, in particular, to correct misinformation. It is also an opportunity to confirm that a woman has accurate information about emergency contraception and how to access it locally.

Contraception should be used from the first act of intercourse as ovulation can occur as early as ten days after an abortion.

- An intrauterine contraceptive device can usually be inserted at the same time as the abortion in the first trimester.
- Depo progestogens can be given prior to discharge from hospital and the oral contraceptive pill can be started immediately after the abortion.
- A diaphragm can usually be fitted after the next menstrual period.
- Natural family planning methods, including Persona are not suitable until regular periods have re-established (usually after two cycles).
- Contraceptive implants can be inserted at the time of abortion if the woman and her doctor are certain of the choice.
- Sterilisation is best done as an interval procedure, both to allow time to come to terms with the abortion and because there may be a small increase in the failure rate when clips are applied to oedematous pregnant fallopian tubes. However in some circumstances, particularly when the decision to have a sterilisation has been made prior to the unplanned pregnancy, sterilisation may be appropriate.

If contraception is not required a woman should be encouraged to have some condoms available, and should know where to go if she requires another method of contraception in the future.

part 12 key message

Fertility control is an important aspect of health care that affects both women and men. Despite modern advances in contraception there will always be unplanned conceptions, and women will always seek abortions whether or not these are legal. The provision of safe early abortion worldwide could save the lives of 70,000[15] women. Abortion is legal in Great Britain but it remains important that it is also accessible to those who most need it. GPs have an important part to play in this access.

part 13 further reading

- ***Abortion services in England and Wales***
  Paintin D (ed) 1994
  Birth Control Trust & British Pregnancy Advisory Service BCT, 1994

- ***Abortion and afterward***
  Davies V
  Ashgrove Press, 1991

- ***Coping with a termination***
  Haslam D
  Cedar Health, 1996

- ***Fetal awareness – report of a Working Party***
  RCOG, 1997

- ***Induced abortion: guideline no. 11***
  RGOC, 1997

- ***Modern methods of inducing abortion***
  Baird DT, Grimes DA and Van Look P (eds)
  Blackwell Science, 1995

- ***The prevention of pelvic infection***
  Templeon A (ed)
  'Prophylactic antibiotic therapy for abortion'
  Penney GC
  RCOG, 1996

- ***Pregnancy and abortion counselling***
  Brien J and Fairbain I
  Routledge, 1996

- ***Pregnancy loss and the death of a baby – guidelines for professionals***
  Kohner N
  Stillbirth and Neonatal Death Society (SANDS), 1995

- ***Report of the RCOG Working Party on Unplanned Pregnancy***
  RCOG, 1991

- ***Under 16s – the law and public policy on contraception and abortion in the UK***
  Brook Advisory Centres, 1995

- ***Unplanned pregnancy: your choices***
  Furedi A
  Oxford University Press, 1996

- ***Unplanned pregnancy – making the right choice for you***
  Debby Klein D and Kaufmann T
  2nd edn, Penguin, 1996

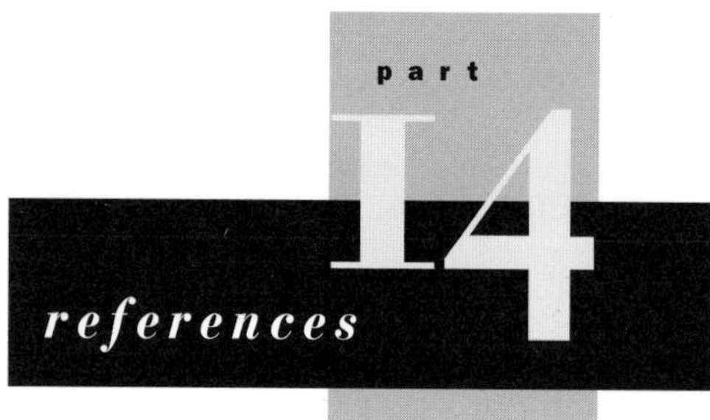

part 14 references

1 ***Population and Health Monitor,*** Series AB, no 96/5, Office for National Statistics, 1996

1a ***Under 16s – the law and public policy on contraception and abortion in the UK,*** Brook Advisory Centres, 1995

2 'Reflex responses do not necessarly signify pain', Lloyd-Thomas AR and Fitzgerald M, ***British Medical Journal, 313,*** 1996, 797-98

3 'Comparison of medical abortion with surgical vacuum aspiration: women's preferences and acceptability of treatment', Henshaw RC, Naji SA and Russell IT, et al, ***British Medical Journal, 307*** 1993, 714-17

4 'What do women want during medical abortion?', Thong KJ, Dewar MH and Baird DT, ***Contraception, 46,*** 1992, 435-42

5 'Antigestogens', Baird DT, 1993, ***British Medical Bulletin, 49,*** 1993, 1,73-87

6 'WHO Task force on post ovulatory methods of fertility regulation', ***British Medical Journal, 307*** 1993, 532-37

7 'Induction of abortion with mifepristone and oral or vaginal misoprostol', El-Refaey H, Rajasekar D and Abdalla M, et al, ***New England Journal of Medicine, 332,*** 1995, 983-87

8 'An effective low cost regime for early medical abortion', Penney GC, McKessock L and Rispin R, et al, ***British Journal of Family Planning, 21,*** 1995, 5-6

9 'Cervical priming with prostaglandin E1 analogue, misopostol and gemeprost' El-Refaey H, Calder L and Wheatley DN, et al, ***The Lancet, 343,*** 1994, 1206-7 (erratum p1650)

10 'Antibiotics at the time of induced abortion: the case for universal prophylaxix based on a meta-analysis', Sawaya GF, Grady D and Kerlikowske, et al, ***Obstetrics and Gynaecology, 87,*** 1996, 884-90

11 'Early complications after induced first trimester abortion', Heisterberg L and Kringelbach M, ***Acta Obstetrica et Gynaecologica, Scandanavia, 66,*** 1987, 201-204

12 'Abortions that fail', Kaunitz AM, Rovira EZ and Grimes DA, ***Obstetrics and Gynaecology, 66,*** 1985, 533-37

13 'The psychological sequelae of theraputic abortion – denied and completed', Dagg PKB, ***American Journal of Psychiatry, 148,*** 1991, 578-85

14 'Termination of pregnancy and psychiatric morbidity', Gilchrist AC, Hannaford PC and Frank P, et al ***British Journal of Psychiatry, 167,*** 1995, 243-48

15 ***Abortion: a tabulation of available data of the frequency and mortality of unsafe abortion,*** Maternal Health and Safe Motherhood Program, 2nd edition, Geneva WHO Division of Family Health, 1993

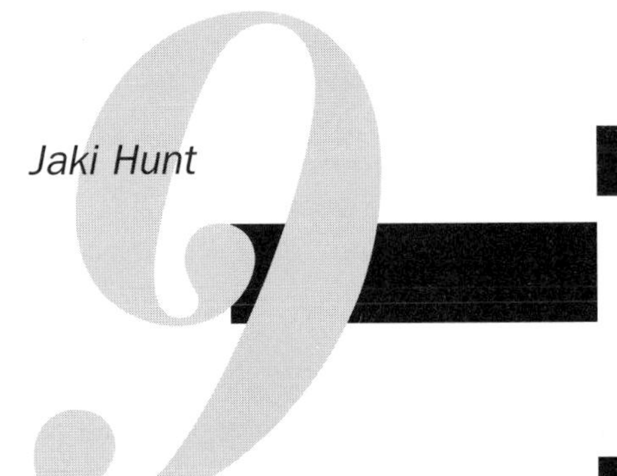

Jaki Hunt

chapter nine

sexually transmitted infections

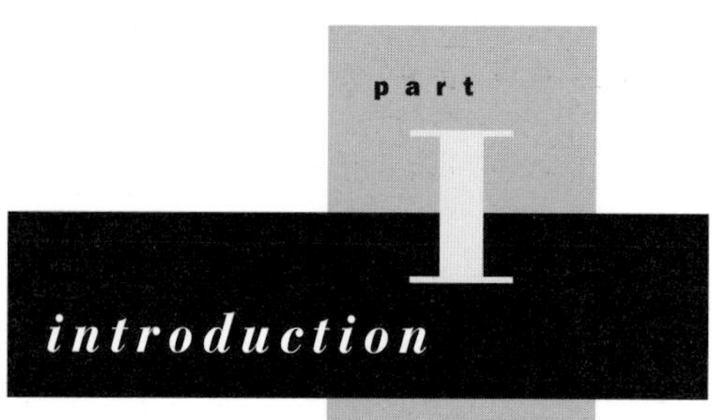

part 1 introduction

Sexually transmitted infections (STIs) are common, particularly among sexually active young people. Their long term sequelae can pose serious health risks, including infertility. In some cases they are life threatening. It is therefore vital to prevent them if possible, and, if not, to detect and treat them early.

STIs create a number of difficulties in primary care, as they may present either with or without symptoms. Primary presentations usually take the form of irritation, discharge (vaginal or urethral), lumps or ulcers (see Table 1, page 135). Secondary STI presentations in general practice include pelvic inflammatory disease (PID), pelvic pain, infertility, cervical dysplasia and miscarriage, ectopic pregnancy or premature labour. The seroconversion illness of HIV may also first present to GPs, although infrequently. Finally, to confuse the picture, some patients will offer a symptom of potential infection to raise worries about their partner's fidelity or fears of HIV.

As a further complication, where one STI has been found others may co-exist. Treatment needs to include screening tests for other infections, along with contact tracing (both to protect the patient from a recurrence, and to protect the community from further spread). Education and health promotion are also important.

It is difficult to know how much of the work should be done in primary care and how much in the genitourinary medicine (GUM) clinic. General practices may feel ill equipped to undertake the full range of tasks. The GUM clinic can be very useful as it has the staff and skills to handle problems, diagnoses and contact tracing quickly and efficiently. However many patients are too embarrassed or frightened to go to the GUM clinic, so it is important to be confident about what good practice is possible in the surgery.

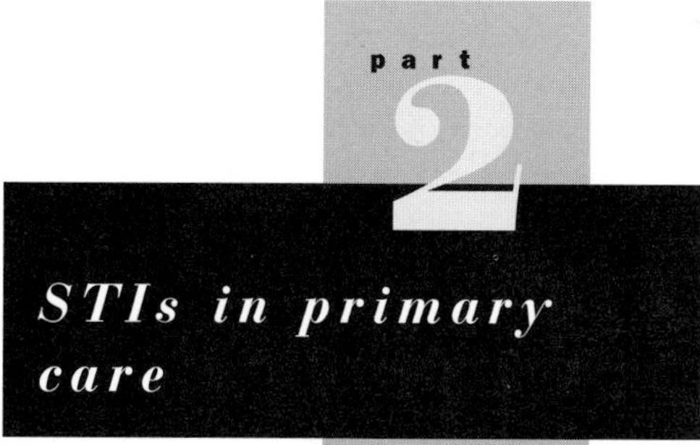

part 2 STIs in primary care

STIs present to the primary health care team in a multitude of ways – and in multitudes! Suspicions should always be close to the surface, as some patients will be too embarrassed to mention infection directly, or to share their suspected risk with you. It is important to remember that vaginal discharge is not all caused by candida. For a sexually active woman presenting with recurrent discharge, repeat prescriptions for an anti-candidal without an accurate diagnosis is not the best response. Even if candida is found, other infections may co-exist or there may be an underlying problem that allows candida access.

Table 1. Common STI presentations in the UK

Primary presentations	Secondary presentations
irritation	sterile pyuria
dysuria	pelvic pain and dyspareunia
discharge (vaginal or urethral)	peri-hepatitis and peri-appendicitis
lumps	menstrual irregularities and breakthrough bleeding
ulcers (painful or non-painful)	cervical smear abnormalities
testicular or epididymal pain	miscarriage
	ectopic pregnancy
	premature labour
	conjunctivitis
	reactive arthritis

HIV, AIDS and Hepatitis B can also present in primary care.

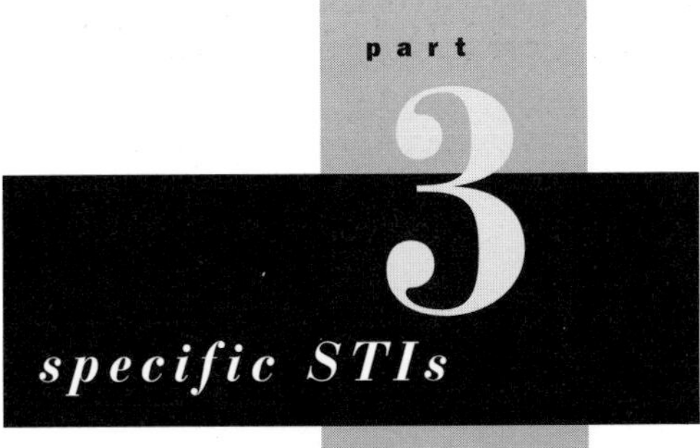

The following section gives a brief resume, of the common STIs in the UK, with their possible presentations in primary care and the risks they carry if not treated.

Chlamydia

Chlamydia trachomatis is the most common bacterial STI in the UK (124 new cases per 100,000 population aged 15-64 were identified in English GUM clinics in 1995; many more will have presented in primary care[1]). It can be asymptomatic in up to 70 per cent of women and more than 50 per cent of men, creating a 'reservoir' of unknown infection amongst the sexually active population. This can only be treated if uncovered, by either contact tracing or screening. Prevalence differs enormously between different populations – 10 per cent in one study, 1 to 2 per cent in others[1a]. Each general practice may have to find out how much chlamydia they have, before deciding how high their level of suspicion should be.

Symptoms, if present, may be of discharge (urethral or, occasionally, vaginal) or dysuria in both genders, of menstrual abnormalities or pelvic pain in women and of testicular pain or discomfort (epididymitis) in men. Reactive arthritis can occur in both men and women. Chlamydial PID in women is a major cause of infertility and ectopic pregnancy in the UK, with these risks increasing with recurrent infection[2]. It is also a cause of chronic pelvic pain, dyspareunia and menstrual disturbances, often with no preceding symptoms of infection, and may have been caught many years before. The disease may also present with infections in the neonate – conjunctivitis that does not respond to standard treatment, or pneumonia.

Treatment is with a tetracycline (eg doxycycline 100mg twice a day for 7 to 14 days), erythromycin (500mg twice a day for 14 days) or a single dose of azithromycin (1 gm stat). (Some of these drugs may also be used to treat gonorrhoea, but swabs would need to be taken for sensitivities.) If treated early (within 3-6 days of first symptoms) there is a much reduced risk of long term tubal damage[3]. This presents a major challenge to primary care, both to prevent initial infection, and to diagnose and treat early (on suspicion, even before tests confirm the diagnosis) if it is found. It also raises issues of screening, particularly before invasive procedures such as termination of pregnancy and IUD insertion[4] (see Chapters 4 and 6) or of at-risk populations[5].

Gonorrhoea

Neisseria gonorrhoeae infection rates fell dramatically in the UK between the 1970s and 1994, but recent figures show that they are now increasing again (overall, 39 per 100,000 population aged 15-64, diagnosed in English GUM clinics in 1995[1]). Although its prevalence in the UK is lower than that of chlamydia, it still causes preventable disease.

The infection is now producing less marked symptoms than in the past, and may even be asymptomatic. However, male symptoms are typically of discharge and/or dysuria (dysuria alone can be a presentation in primary care), and female symptoms are of discharge, dysuria or abdominal pain.

In women, gonorrhoea carries the risks of PID, infertility and ectopic pregnancy, and these can follow an asymptomatic initial infection. In pregnancy, it can be transmitted to the neonate at delivery (leading to gonococcal ophthalmia neonatorum and the risk of blindness) and can cause postpartum endometritis and pelvic sepsis. In men, gonorrhoea can cause epididymitis.
In UK GUM clinics, it is usually treated with penicillins, or with a single dose of ciprofloxacin (500mg stat) or ofloxacin (400mg stat). It can rapidly develop resistance to drugs that are widely used in a community (eg penicillin), so gonorrhoea caught abroad may have a completely different sensitivity pattern to that caught in the UK. Sensitivities from swabs will assist with the choice of drug, but will delay treatment. The local GUM clinic or microbiology lab should be able to help to choose the 'best guess' option, ahead of these results.

Non specific urethritis (NSU) or non specific genital infection (NSGI)

NSU is a common infection in men in the UK, with 317 per 100,000 population aged 15-64[1], diagnosed in English GUM clinics in 1995. The diagnosis at present is one of exclusion – effectively urethritis that is not caused by gonorrhoea. Up to 40 per cent of NSU is caused by chlamydia, and a number of other infective agents have also been implicated, including Ureaplasma urealyticum and Mycoplasma genitalium.

The usual presentation is in men, with discharge and/or dysuria. Urethritis is the most common cause of dysuria in sexually active young men. Female partners of men infected with non-chlamydial NSU often carry the bacteria without symptoms, but may still incur health risks[6]. As treating female partners also reduces the risk of NSU recurrence in men[7], it is important to trace and treat sexual contacts.

In the GUM clinic, diagnosis is made from an intraurethral swab, showing 5 or more pus cells per high power field (x400) in the absence of gonorrhoea. In primary care, where microscopy is not readily available, swabs should be sent for both chlamydial and bacterial culture, but may well be negative. Pus cells can be markers of inflammation as well as infection, and can persist after infection has cleared. Some causes of NSU may be non-infective, possibly caused by urethral irritants. This could explain the rate of recurrence in some men whose only sexual partner has also been treated. Because the persistence of pus cells after infection is possible, post treatment tests of cure can be confusing, and may therefore only be appropriate if symptoms persist.

Treatment is with tetracyclines or erthromycin (as for chlamydia, page 135).

Trichomonas vaginalis

Trichomoniasis is one of the most common STIs world wide, and is most prevalent in developing countries, where it may play a role in the transmission of HIV[8]. Seventeen cases per 100,000 population aged 15-64 were identified in English GUM clinics in 1995[1], so it still remains relevant to our population. The classic symptoms in a woman are of a greenish yellow vaginal discharge (often 'frothy'), accompanied by soreness, itching and dyspareunia, but it can be asymptomatic. Men are often asymptomatic, but can have urethral irritation, dysuria and/or discharge. It is important to treat male partners, even if the organism cannot be found on them, as this reduces reinfection for women[8].

In the GUM clinic, diagnosis is usually made by microscopy of a wet preparation of discharge by an experienced microscopist, although such tests on a male may be negative. In primary care a high vaginal swab is sent for culture or special staining. Treatment of both partners is with metronidazole – either as a 5 day course of 400mg bd, or a single 2 gm dose. Post treatment tests of cure are important to identify treatment failure and reduce recurrence.

Herpes simplex virus (HSV)

The number of episodes of genital herpes simplex seen in GUM clinics has been rising steadily since 1988, with 85 cases per 100,000 population aged 15-64 identified in English GUM clinics in 1995[1]. This figure includes new cases and recurrences. Viral typing demonstrates that both HSV 1 and HSV 2 cause genital attacks, with HSV 2 carrying a higher risk of recurrence and causing more severe disease.

Serological testing shows that up to 70 per cent of people with HSV 2 infections are asymptomatic, and therefore are unknowingly risking transmission of the virus to their partners[9]. Orogenital transmission of herpes is possible from a partner who has cold sores, and can explain the occurrence of a primary episode in a monogamous relationship. Asymptomatic viral shedding can occur in both genital and oral HSV, particularly during the prodrome and after an attack. Susceptible women are more likely to contract the virus from genital contact with an infected partner than men[10], and barrier contraception offers some protection against transmission.

Primary infections cause a systemic 'flu-like prodrome, followed by severe painful genital ulceration. Recurrences may feature local prodromal symptoms such as tingling and discomfort, typically progressing to localised papules, blisters, ulcers and crusting lesions, and can be initiated by a variety of stimuli. Neonatal herpes carries the risk of disability and death to the infant, but is rare in the UK, occurring mainly in the presence of a primary infection around the time of delivery.

Diagnosis is not always straightforward, and may be confirmed by taking viral swabs for HSV from fresh ulcers (an uncomfortable procedure for the patient). The psychological impact of an HSV diagnosis can have major implications for the individual, fuelled by messages from the media. It is therefore important to confirm HSV before giving the patient a disease label that may, to them, sound like a life sentence. It is also vital to have confirmed the diagnosis before prescribing prophylaxis for recurrent symptoms.

Treatment should include symptom control (analgesia, local wound care), stress reduction (rest, relaxation techniques) and patient counselling and support (possibly including help from support groups). Anti-virals (for example aciclovir, famciclovir or valaciclovir) have been shown to ease symptoms if started early in a primary infection (before, or soon after, ulcers develop), and can be used long term to suppress attacks in patients with frequent and severe recurrences. Although there is little evidence to demonstrate the worth of episodic treatment with these drugs, they are sometimes used in this way in GUM clinics. It is not clear whether they reduce transmission of the virus, although they have been shown to reduce viral shedding[11]. The evidence to date does not support using anti-virals to reduce transmission.

Human papilloma virus (HPV) – genital warts

Figures for first presentation of genital warts in GUM clinics are rising (161 per 100,000 population aged 15-64, in 1995[1]). There are many types of genital HPV, falling into two discrete disease-producing groups; those that cause warts and those that are associated with an increased risk of cervical cancer. HPV is very common amongst sexually active young people, often without the presence of visible warts. However, as genital HPV is sexually transmitted, the presence of warts, or of wart virus on cervical cytology, suggests that the patient has been at risk of other STIs.

The treatment of warts is arguably cosmetic, although they can cause a huge amount of distress, and GUM clinicians believe that they are at their most infectious when present as visible lesions. Topical treatment with podophyllin needs to be applied by a health care professional (once or twice a week, with the initial application washed off after four hours to reduce the risk of skin ulceration), but podophyllotoxin can be self applied. Other treatments include hyfrecation and excision.

It is important to take a cervical smear in women presenting with warts[12] (unless they have had one recently), and to inform the laboratory of the presence of warts. (While visible warts do not usually lead to cervical changes, they may indicate the presence of other wart virus which could cause neoplasia.) Follow up cytology at more frequent intervals is not routinely required, and should be based on the smear report.

Bacterial vaginosis (BV)

BV describes a clinical syndrome, where anaerobic bacteria replace the normal vaginal flora (lactobacilli). This can create a foul 'fishy' smelling discharge but is often asymptomatic. Diagnosis is made by looking for the classic thin white/grey vaginal discharge, testing it for pH (positive if greater than 4.5), and getting a positive amine test (releasing a recognisable 'amine' smell after adding a drop of potassium hydroxide). Where microscopy is available, 'clue cells' may be found. The presence of three out of four of these leads to the diagnosis. A high vaginal swab will show the presence of unusual bacteria, often with gardnerella vaginalis, and will also differentiate from trichomonas infection, which can have very similar signs.

BV is often seen in primary care. 290 new cases of 'vaginosis/vaginitis' per 100,000 of the female population aged 15-64 were identified in English GUM clinics in 1995, and these figures will include those for BV. There is dispute as to whether BV is sexually transmitted, and studies show that the treatment of sexual partners does not improve the recurrence rate for women[13].

There is increasing evidence that the infection can cause serious risks in pregnancy. One group found that by eradicating BV in pregnant women, they were able to reduce the rates of pregnancy loss before 22 weeks, premature rupture of membranes and preterm birth[14]. Work is in progress to look at whether it is worthwhile to screen for BV in pregnancy, to define who should be treated and to find the best treatment regimes[15]. However, it is already clear that if medication is used in pregnancy, it needs to be systemic rather than intravaginal, and to be given early (first trimester, if possible). Oral metronidazole or clindamycin vaginal cream are recommended at present, although the high dose regime of metronidazole (2 gm stat) is contraindicated in pregnancy. Dalacin (clindamycin) cream may offer symptomatic relief, but should only be used if pregnancy in the near future is not likely.

Candida

Although Candida albicans is not generally sexually transmitted, it often presents in GUM clinics (219 cases per 100,000 population of men and women aged 15-64, in 1995[1]), and should be treated as part of the spectrum of sexually transmitted infection. Common as it is in primary care, it may occasionally be associated with sexual transmission, or other sexual problems. The classic symptoms in women are a thick white ('cheesy') itchy vaginal discharge, and in men, an itchy penile rash often accompanied by a discharge under the foreskin. The infection is often recurrent, and can cause much distress to the sufferer.

Candida albicans acts as an opportunistic organism, taking advantage of factors that lower the host's immune defences[16]. Such factors include immune deficiencies (eg HIV disease, use of immunosuppressive therapy), endocrine diseases (for example diabetes mellitus), pregnancy, malignancy, post radiation therapy, local allergens and other STIs. Although evidence shows that the older high dose oestrogen oral contraceptive predisposed to candidal infection, it is not thought that modern low dose pills do[17]. Broad spectrum antibiotics encourage candidal colonisation.

Treatment of recurrent attacks should include reviewing the possibility of underlying reduction in host resistance alongside the sustained use of anti-fungals, possibly prophylactically, in order to prevent recurrences. Treatment of male partners with local anti-fungals may prevent the reintroduction of the organism in recurrent cases, but the mainstay of treatment remains the use of anti-fungal treatment for the symptomatic patient.

Syphilis

New cases of syphilis are rare in the UK (4.5 cases per 100,000 population for all syphilis and 0.9 cases per 100,000 population for infectious syphilis in GUM clinics in 1995[1]). Most of these cases will have been discovered as a result of serology taken for screening (eg in pregnancy or for blood donation) and in the absence of symptoms. Expertise is needed to decide whether treatment and contact tracing is needed, so referral to the local GUM clinic or microbiologist is important.

Viral hepatitis

Hepatitis B is a sexually transmitted infection, and is more infectious than HIV. 2.2 new antigen positive cases per 100,000 population were reported in GUM clinics in 1995[1]. Antigen testing and vaccination are available to people at risk of catching this infection (health care professionals, partners of infected patients, sexually active homosexual men and drug users who share injecting equipment). Some countries are offering routine vaccination to children. Specialised units in the UK offer advice and treatment options to patients.

Hepatitis A can be caught sexually when partners have acute infection. Vaccination is now available, either on its own or in a combination with hepatitis B vaccine.

Pubic lice

Although not a sexually transmitted infection in their own right, these co-exist with STIs and their presence should alert one to the need to consider the possibility of infection with one of the others. Treatment is as for head lice. There may be a locally recommended treatment because of resistance problems.

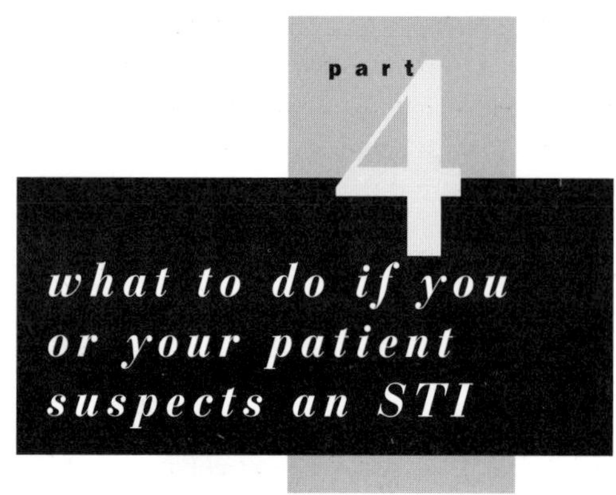

Take a sexual history

Taking a sexual history is covered in Chapter 2. It is important to include direct questions about partners, both to assess risk, and to trace contacts if an infection is found. Do not make assumptions about the gender of a partner in your questions. A patient who was thinking of revealing his homosexuality (and his fear of HIV) to you is unlikely to do so if you ask

'Have you got a girlfriend at the moment?'

or

'How many women have you slept with?'.

A more open question –

'Do you have a sexual partner at the moment?'

– is more likely to allow an honest answer.

It is worth remembering that some patients use a symptom of potential infection as a 'ticket of admission', to invite you to open doors onto their fears and secrets. Recent or past sexual abuse can be uncovered in this context, as can a range of psychosexual problems (see Chapter 10). The symptom still needs to be investigated, but so does the underlying distress.

Refer to a GUM clinic if the patient agrees

Suggest that if the patient agrees, s/he can be referred to a GUM clinic. Explain that as specialist centres, they have comprehensive facilities for treating STIs. GUM clinics accept self-referrals, or referrals from any member of the primary health care team. If the local clinic runs an appointment system, a time can usually be arranged over the telephone. Most clinics can 'fit in' urgent appointments, particularly if requested by a health care professional. Some clinics run an open access system, allowing patients to turn up without an appointment. Because GUM clinics guarantee confidentiality to their patients, they are unlikely to write after a patient has self-referred to them. However, if a referrer has written a letter, they will usually reply.

If the patient is referred to the GUM clinic for tests, it is preferable not to start drug treatment in advance, as it can destroy 'the evidence'. This decision may be influenced by the potential waiting time for a clinic appointment, or by a belief that the patient will not attend.

GUM clinics will often be able to make a diagnosis at the first visit, and can supply treatment without a prescription charge. Their health adviser will tackle contact tracing, and can network with other clinics nationally to follow this up. Some patients feel more able to be honest about their contacts in the confidential and private atmosphere of a clinic.

However, some patients dread the idea of attending a GUM clinic, expecting to find the waiting room full of either local gossips or prostitutes! This may reflect their own feelings about sex and STIs ('dirty', 'disgusting'). Some clinics now run 'sexual health' clinics, offering family planning and psychosexual medicine alongside GU medicine, which can help patients to feel more comfortable. It can also help if the referrer knows how the clinic runs, and can transmit positive messages to the patient when discussing the need for referral. A professional visit to the local clinic could, therefore, be very useful for anyone planning to refer patients there.

Although most patients will attend a GUM clinic if the advantages are explained, there will always be some who prefer to be treated in general practice. If these guidelines are followed, the work can be done well in primary care.

Make an accurate diagnosis

*For **women**, tests for STIs should include:*

- endocervical swab for gonorrhoea (do first – taking the discharge)
- endocervical swab for chlamydia (get cells with a vigorous rotatory motion in the cervical canal for best result)
- vaginal swab for trichomonas, gardnerella and candida (anterior fornix is best)
- vaginal pH (dip litmus paper in discharge on swab or slide)
- amine test (put discharge on slide, add drop of potassium hydroxide and sniff)

and could include:

- viral swabs for herpes following the advice of your local laboratory (these tests differ between labs)
- cervical smear – if she is not up to date with screening[12], if the cervix looks suspicious or in the presence of warts
- blood tests for syphilis and HIV with appropriate counselling. Remember that it can take up to three months (the 'window period') before these tests become positive
- microscopy of vaginal discharge for clue cells, trichomonas and candida
- if gonorrhoea is suspected, swabs from the mouth and rectum should also be taken

*For **men**, tests for STIs should include:*

- urethral swabs for gonorrhoea
- urethral swabs for chlamydia (or a first void urine test if locally available)
- microscopy of urethral smear for NSU

and could include:

- swabs from the sub-prepuce to look for candida
- proctoscopy and rectal swabs in men who have had receptive anal sex
- blood tests for syphilis and HIV. Again, remember the window period and offer counselling
- If gonorrhoea is suspected, swabs from the mouth and rectum should also be taken

Microscopy of samples can allow an immediate diagnosis of NSU in men and of trichomonas, gonorrhoea, and candida in both men and women. NSU may be missed without microscopy of male urethral samples. Apart from the few practices that have a microscope and someone who can use it, this option is not available in general practice.

Discussion with the pathology lab will help to decide which tests should be kept in stock, what training is needed to take them and what their transport and storage requirements are. There may be large differences in the samples needed for these tests by different laboratories. The sensitivity and specificity of the results will also differ between labs.

Sensitivity and specificity will be greatly affected by transport to the laboratory, and storage in the practice. Ensure that samples go straight into the fridge, and do not hang about until the surgery is finished, and that they go straight from the fridge to the transport, without warming up.

Tests must be taken before embarking on treatment, because it may be impossible to make a diagnosis afterwards. A 'best guess' treatment after tests have been taken will often be appropriate, but should be reviewed once the results are back.

Offer tests for other STIs

As STIs can coexist, when one infection is found it is appropriate to test for others. Patients may have a secret fear of HIV, so the option of this test could also be offered.

Treat infections

A number of factors need to be considered when choosing a treatment regime. The ideal treatment choice would offer 100 per cent bacterial sensitivity and cure rates, be free from side effects, be taken in a single dose or a short course, and carry no potential risks to a fetus (some women may be unknowingly pregnant after unprotected intercourse). Compliance is an important issue, as many patients will forget their treatment once symptoms have settled. For this reason, single dose regimes are often now used in UK GUM clinics although they are more expensive than the traditional longer courses.

Appropriate treatments for the various diagnoses are specified in Part 3 (pages 135 – 139). However, the local pathology lab or GUM clinic may advise on local resistance problems.

While taking treatment, patients should be advised either to abstain from sexual intercourse (this is not always a practical option, and some patients may lose respect for you if you insist) or to use a condom. This is to avoid passing the infection on, and to prevent reinfection from a partner who has not yet completed their own treatment. For some infections (see below), this should be continued until a negative 'test of cure' has been achieved for both partners.

Test for cure if needed

'Tests of cure' should be taken after treatment

- for gonorrhoea – because of the possibility of drug resistance
- for trichomonas – because treatment failures occur

'Tests of cure' need not be taken after treatment unless symptoms persist, reinfection is possible, or the treatment was not completed

- for chlamydia – there is good evidence that the infection has not developed resistance to today's drugs[18], and it can take up to four weeks for the test to become negative after an infection is treated
- for vaginal candida unless recurrent
- for bacterial vaginosis – though it may reassure the patient, and identify the occasional case of resistance

Discuss future problems and follow up

Some patients will have heard of the sequelae of STIs – for instance, the risks to fertility of chlamydia and gonorrhoea, and the association of warts with cervical cancer. The details may be misunderstood, leading to inappropriate fears. Patients need time to express their worries, to receive appropriate health education and to sort out future follow up (eg appropriate cervical smears after genital warts have been found).

Contact trace and treat

It is important to trace, test and treat the sexual partners of a patient with an STI. Reinfection of the patient is highly likely if their partner continues to carry the infection and further community spread of the infection can be reduced by treating contacts. Completing this task can be very complicated, as an accurate diagnosis is needed in each case to decide whether the contacts of the contact should also be involved. Many general practices will feel that this is beyond their capabilities, especially when contacts are not patients of the practice. Fortunately, the local GUM clinic is well placed to do the work, steering through the complexities of geography, confidentiality and distrust that are often present.

Maintain confidentiality

Confidentiality is important to patients with an STI. Unless they have trust and can expect complete privacy, they may not reveal their full story. Patients may have general concerns about confidentiality in general practices[19], and this will be heightened with STIs. This is particularly true for younger patients, who may be frightened even of being seen at the surgery at a time when their parents don't know about their visit. They may see practice staff as family friends, and therefore expect information to be passed on to their neighbours and parents. These misconceptions can make it very difficult for some patients to be honest about their symptoms and fears to their GP. Practices may wish to address this issue, for example with public notices about confidentiality in the waiting room (see Chapter 3, page 57).

Educate

A patient in whom an STI is suspected is a prime candidate for sexual health promotion. This is an ideal time to discuss risky behaviour, answer questions about sexual health, and raise relevant issues that they may not be aware of. This is also a good time to encourage patients to discuss safer sex with their partner, to insist on a condom in the future, or even to say 'No' next time. Each patient will have a different balance of need, be it practical ('What's the best way of putting on a condom?'), educational ('What's the risk of HIV?') or emotional ('He'll leave me if I say "No"'). This may be an area where the skills of the practice nurse could be put to good use.

Check contraceptive needs

If there has been the risk of acquiring an STI, then it is possible that there has also been the risk of pregnancy. Along with discussion of 'Double Dutch' contraception methods (the condom alongside the pill, for example), this could be a good time to review family planning for this patient, or even to introduce them to it (see Chapter 6).

Support and counsel

An STI diagnosis can powerfully destroy the trust within a relationship – not always appropriately. It may reawaken the distress of previous betrayals or attacks (including childhood sexual abuse) or bring other 'secrets' close to the surface (for example uncertainty about sexuality). Feelings of disgust, guilt, or anger may overwhelm the patient and the very practical need to tell contacts of their own risks can be emotionally difficult to tackle. The future risks from this infection and the possibilities of others may need airing, along with underlying fears of HIV.

A non-judgemental and open approach is vital. Careful work now could protect the patient from future physical risks, and prevent this experience from initiating or exacerbating a psychosexual problem (see Chapter 10). This will take time and skill, but could help a patient to improve their life dramatically.

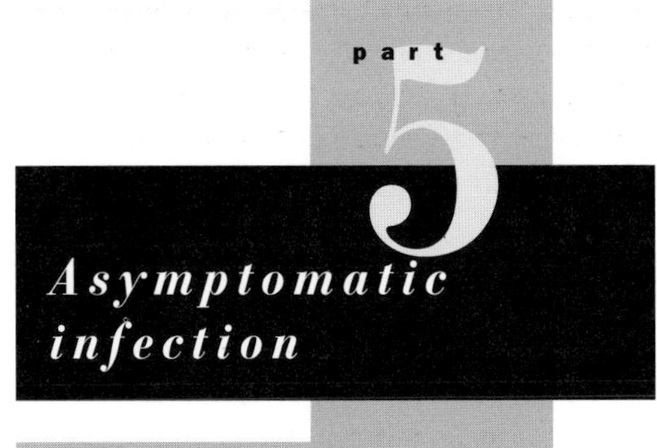

Asymptomatic infection

Asymptomatic infections may present to primary care in a number of ways.

A patient may have received a 'contact slip' (issued by a GUM clinic) from a partner or through the post. This contains a code identifying the partner's infection which can be decoded by the local GUM clinic (See *'A guide to GUM codes'*, page 144). Inform the issuing GUM clinic if you deal with this presentation within the practice, in order to help them to monitor their contact tracing.

Both chlamydia and gonorrhoea can initially be asymptomatic in women, only revealing themselves when the sequelae of PID or infertility are discovered. These infections can be transferred from the vagina to the fallopian tubes by an invasive procedure such as fitting an IUD[4]. As 10 per cent of sexually active women may be infected with chlamydia, it is appropriate to screen for chlamydia before IUD insertion, and then either to give a presumptive single dose treatment (eg azithromycin 1gm) or to await results. If infection is found, treat the patient, test her contact and advise condom use or abstention until both are infection free. (National guidelines are pending.)

Asymptomatic wart virus infection can present on cervical cytology. The HPV types that are associated with cancer do not usually produce warts, but can act as a pointer towards STI risk factors. A patient with such an abnormal smear should therefore be offered an STI screen.

Bacterial vaginosis is often asymptomatic. Recent evidence about possible dangers in pregnancy (see page 138) raises questions about antenatal screening. Work is still being done to find practical answers.

A final group of asymptomatic patients are the 'worried well'. Partner infidelity, local rumours or media interest in a particular infection may have aroused their fears, or they may want to check that all is well before embarking on a new sexual relationship. A full (and negative) STI screen may be all that is needed, although further counselling and support could be necessary. This could also be a good time for sexual health promotion, or discussion of contraception and future fertility.

A guide to GUM codes on STI clinic contact slips

A1-9	**Syphilis (various forms)**
B1-5	**Gonorrhoea (various forms)**
C1-3	**Chancroid and Donovanosis**
C4A-E	**Chlamydia (various types)**
C4H-I	**NSU/NSI/NSGI**
C5	**Complicated non-gonoccal or non - specific infection**
C6A	**Trichomoniasis**
C6B-C	**Bacterial vaginosis/anaerobic infection**
C7A	**Candida**
C8-9	**Scabies/Pediculosis**
C10A-B	**Herpes simplex**
C11 A-C	**Anogenital warts**
C12	**Molluscum contagiosum**
C13-14	**Hepatitis**
D2A	**Urinary tract infection**
D2B-3	**Other conditions**
E1-2	**HIV**
E3	**AIDS**

The 1990 Government White Paper, *The Health of the Nation,* set targets for reducing the incidence of STIs and their sequelae in our population, driven by the dangers of HIV. The ongoing relationship that practices have with their patients and communities allows opportunities for education and sexual health promotion, screening and early diagnosis, and correct treatment and contact tracing. Each of these has a place in preventing future disease.

part 7 key messages

- Refer to GUM clinic if patient agrees
- Take a sexual history, remembering the possibility of rape or sexual abuse
- Make a specific diagnosis by testing for the range of STIs
- Treat all infections found
- Test for cure if needed, particularly in gonorrhoea
- Discuss any potential future problems, and arrange follow up care
- Test and treat partner/s – or arrange for this to be done
- Maintain patient confidentiality throughout
- Educate about prevention, risky behaviour, safer sex and HIV
- Check family planning needs
- Support and counsel

- ***A GP's guide to genitourinary medicine and sexual health***
  Sonnex C
  Cambridge University Press, 1996

- ***The ABC of sexually transmitted diseases***
  Adler M (ed)
  BMJ Publishing Group, 1995

- ***A colour atlas of sexually transmitted disease***
  Wisdom A
  Wolfe Medical Publications, 1995

1 Sexually transmitted diseases, England 1995, new cases seen at NHS genitourinary medicine clinics, ***Statistical Bulletin,*** Department of Health, 14, 1996

1a 'General practice update: chlamydia infection in women', Oakeshott P and Hay P, ***British Journal of General Practice, 45,*** 1995, 615-20; 'Genital chlamydia trachomatis Ross JDC, et al, ***British Medical Journal, 313,*** 1996, 1192-93; 'Epidemiology of genital Chlamydia trachomatis in England and Wales', Simms I, et al, ***Genitourinary Medicine 73,*** 1997, 122-26; 'Chlamydia infection in UK family planning clinics', Stokes T, ***British Journal of Family Planning, 23,*** 1997, 47-50

2 'Pelvic inflammatory disease and fertility', Westrom R, Joesoef R and Reynolds G, et al, ***Sexually Transmitted Diseases, 19,*** 1992,185-92

3 'Delayed care of pelvic inflammatory disease as a risk factor for impaired fertility', Hillis SD, Joesoef R and Marchbanks PA, et al, ***American Journal of Obstetrics and Gynecology, 168*** 1993, 1503-09

4 'Screening for and treating ChlamydiaTrachomatis and Neisseria Gonorrhoea before contraceptive use and subsequent pelvic inflammatory infection', Sprague DS, Bullbough CHW and Rashid S, et al, ***British Journal of Family Planning, 16*** 1990, 54-58

5 'Prevention of pelvic inflammatory disease by screening for cervical chlamydial infection', Scholes D, Stergachis A and Heidrich FE, et al, ***New England Journal of Medicine, 334*** 1996, 1362-66

6 'Infections due to species of Mycoplasma and Ureaplasma: an update', Taylor-Robinson D, ***Clinical Infectious Diseases, 23*** 1996, 671-84

7 'Epidemiological treatment of sexual contacts prevents recurrence of non-gonococcal urethritis', Woolley PD, Wilson JD and Kinghorn GR, et al, ***Genitourinary Medicine, 63*** 1987, 384-85

8 'Trichomonas treatment in women. The Cochrane Database of Systematic Reviews', Gulmezoglu AM, ***Tropical Diseases Module*** 1996

9 'The frequency of unrecognised type 2 herpes simplex virus infection among women', Koutsky LA, Ashley RL and Holmes KK, et al, ***Sexually Transmitted Diseases, 17*** 1990, 90-94

10 'Risk factors for the sexual transmission of genital herpes', Mertz GJ, Benedetti J and Ashley R, et al, ***Annals of Internal Medicine, 116*** 1992, 197-202

11 'Suppression of subclinical shedding of herpes simplex virus type 2 with aciclovir' Wald A, Zeh J, and Barnum G, et al, ***Annals of Internal Medicine, 124,*** 1996, (1 pt 1), 8-15

12 ***Guidelines for clinical practice and programme management: NHS cervical screening programme*** Duncan I, National Co-ordinating Network, Oxford RHA, 1992

13 'Bacterial vaginosis: review of treatment options and potential clinical indications for therapy', Joesoef MR and Schmid GP, ***Clinical Infectious Diseases, 20*** 1995, (Supplement 1) S72-S79

14 'Prevention of premature birth by screening and treatment for common genital tract infections: results of a prospective controlled evaluation', McGregor JA, Freud JI and Panker R, et al, ***American Journal Obstetrics and Gynecology, 173,*** 1995,157-167

15 'Abnormal bacterial colonisation of the genital tract and subsequent preterm delivery and late miscarriage', Hay PE, Lamont RF and Taylor Robinson D, et al, ***British Medical Journal, 308,*** 1994, 295-298

16 'Immunologic factors influencing susceptibility to recurrent candidal vaginitis', Witkin SS, ***Clinical Obstetrics and Gynaecology, 34,*** 1991, 662-68

17 'Management of genital candidiasis', Working Group of the British Society for Medical Mycology, ***British Medical Journal, 310,*** 1995, 1241-1244

18 'Is a test of cure necessary following infection with Chlamydia trachomatis?' Radcliffe K, Raven D, and Mercey D, et al, ***Genitourinary Medicine, 66,*** 1990, 444-46

19 'Sexual health services in Northamptonshire: what do our young people think of them?', Hunt J, Audit project report, Northamptonshire MAAG, 1995

Acknowledgements

I am grateful to Dr Graz Luzzi, Consultant Physician in Genito-urinary Medicine at Wycombe Hospital for his helpful advice and constructive criticism in the preparation of this chapter.

Jaki Hunt

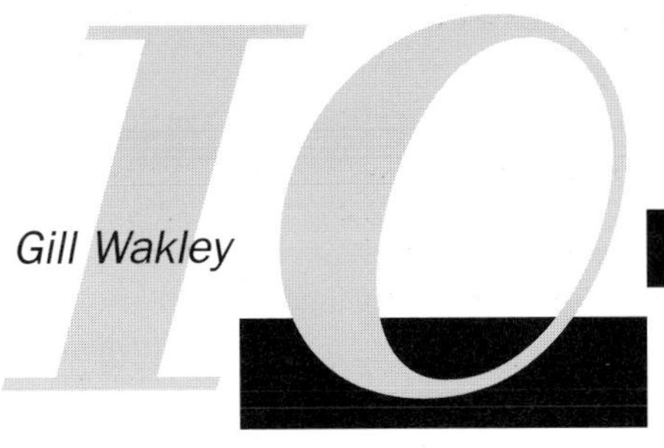

Gill Wakley

chapter ten

sexual problems in primary care

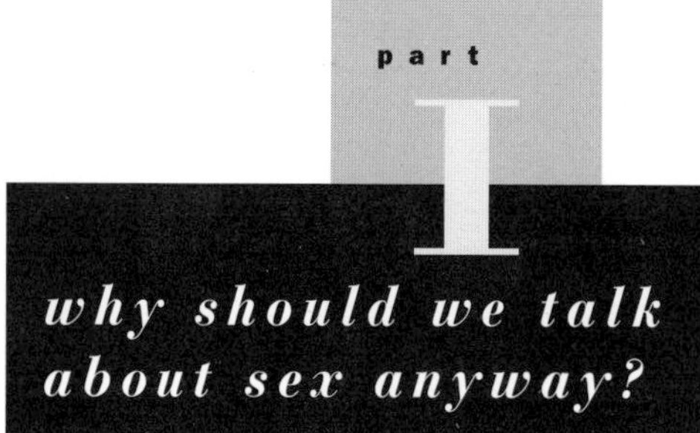

why should we talk about sex anyway?

Primary care is the first port of call for any patient with a problem. It is accessible to all and the reason for attendance is not obvious to others. The prevalence of sexual problems in the general population is uncertain. A study in Oxford, of middle-aged women with partners, showed a prevalence of current dysfunction of 33 per cent[1]. A recent study in several general practices found current rates of 44 per cent for men and 36 per cent for women – a significant number of people with sexual dysfunction[2].

Doctors and nurses need to be competent and willing to hear about sexual problems:

- If you miss the sexual problem you will give the wrong advice or treatment, eg investigating a woman who wants to become pregnant but has non-consummation!
- Your patients may not take important treatment, eg medication for hypertension or depression
- Much unnecessary treatment can be avoided by understanding why patients present with somatic symptoms when they do
- Primary care recognises the need to care for the whole patient including their sexuality
- Patients expect some degree of expertise from health professionals, eg why they get sore after making love
- Expectations of having a satisfactory sexual life have risen and with them, increasing openness about talking about sexuality
- Patients think contraception has something to do with sexual activity and talk about sex more freely[3]
- Health promotion activities such as cervical screening or testicular self-examination, provide natural opening gambits for broaching concerns about sexuality
- Recognition of the importance of the prevention of sexually transmitted infections such as chlamydia should make health professionals proactive in asking about sexual behaviour

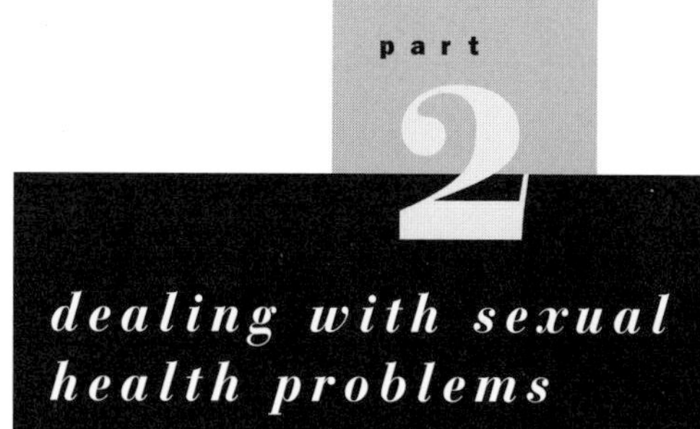

dealing with sexual health problems

Creating the right atmosphere

Sex is often difficult to talk about. It is usually a private concern, alluded to by innuendo and non-verbal signals. Consultation skills are used to elicit the patient's problem (See *Consultation skills for sexual problems* below and Chapter 2).

Sexual problems may be accompanied by reticence and embarrassment on the part of health professional and patient[4].

We have already learnt to ask embarrassing questions ('Have you had your bowels open?' or 'How many days does your period last?') that would not be acceptable in ordinary conversation. We need to recognise our own defences against talking about sexuality in the same matter-of-fact way.

The duty to care for the whole patient

- Doctors and nurses have knowledge about and some responsibility for, the bodies of their patients
- The doctor or nurse who uses psychodynamic skills, but who wishes to treat the whole person, cannot forget the traditional skills of

physical doctoring or nursing
- Study both the emotional and the physical aspects. It provides an understanding of how the whole person functions
- Recognise that patients have the information within themselves that can enable them to resolve their sexual problems in a way that will suit them best. The doctor or nurse does not need to be an expert at sexual problems, just an expert at helping patients
- We should not offer reassurance or advice before the problem is understood by both the patient and the health professional
- Recognise your own limitations and those of the patient. Refer those beyond your capabilities. Do not continue to offer help and time to those patients who cannot use them constructively

If you ask a lot of questions you get a lot of answers – but you may not hear what the problem is because you have not allowed the patient to tell you. Closed questions make sure that the patient stays closed off too!

Health professionals are very privileged to be able to look at the bodies of their patients unclothed and revealed. Imagine what a patient would say if asked to undress by a marriage guidance counsellor! The doctor needs to listen and observe during the physical examination, not just find or exclude physical abnormalities. The vulnerability of patients during physical examination often enables them to make connections between the complaint and the feelings.

CONSULTATION SKILLS FOR SEXUAL PROBLEMS

- **Using how the patient makes you feel to illustrate or interpret how the patient may relate to others[5]**
- **Noticing and using non-verbal communication**
- **Tolerating not knowing what to do[6]**
- **Recognising your own biases and prejudices**
- **Having some knowledge of sexual functioning and emotional development[7]**
- **Using the physical examination as an exploration of the emotional and physical factors[8]**
- **Giving advice or reassurance only when the doctor has checked that the problem is understood**
- **Recognising when to refer elsewhere**
- **Recognising when to limit offers of help**

Dealing with the information about sexuality

Sexual difficulties may be:
- discovered as part of an on-going illness, or as a side effect of treatment
- presented openly
- presented after a visiting card of a related (or even unrelated) complaint
- hidden by a psychosomatic complaint

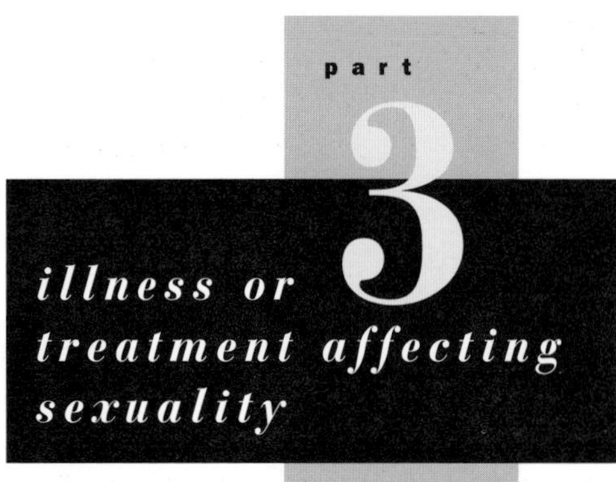

Loss of interest in sexual activity while ill is common. The results of long term illness can be divided into three sections – but each has its effect on the other.

The psychological effects of being ill

Individuals may feel sexually unattractive, embarrassed by how they look, or that they are not worth bothering about. Relationships change – a man or woman previously active and having a definite role, becomes reliant on others and more childlike. Sex seems not appropriate, or even wrong, in this child-adult relationship. The couple may feel that sexual activity may damage the sufferer, or that the excitement of orgasm will be harmful.

The physical effects of being ill

Nerve or blood vessel damage directly affect the genitals, other erogenous zones or hormone levels. Pain, loss of flexibility and mobility, being too fat or too thin, all make sexual activity difficult or so painful that it is avoided even if desire is present.

The effect of treatment

Drugs may make the suffers drowsy, or too tired to bother, or cause direct effects on the erection or the orgasm. Surgery may damage the genital organs or remove part of the body that the sufferer feels is necessary to their sexuality. Treatment can also result in scarring or disfigurement, leading to loss of self-esteem.

See Table 1: *Common problems leading to sexual difficulties* (page 154).

Painful sex: a common problem

WOMEN

- Failure of arousal may cause pain on intercourse
- Psychological problems are the usual cause of vaginismus, but can be secondary to dyspareunia
- Rarely, the hymen is thick and tough and prevents penetration
- Infections of the vagina will cause pain, and the vaginal walls are tender and less well lubricated during the recovery from an infection
- Similar problems of tender scar tissue may occur after any stitching of the vulva or vagina
- The Bartolin's glands may become infected, or develop cystic swelling, causing local pain
- The ballooning of the vagina and pulling up of the uterus will not occur without sexual arousal and deep pain from impact on the tissues and cervix will further inhibit response
- Infection of the tubes, and conditions such as endometriosis, may cause pain on deep thrusting
- A tender or distended bowel, common in conditions such as the irritable bowel syndrome or diverticular disease, can inhibit responsiveness
- Constant pelvic pain that persists after negative investigations may be linked to changes in blood flow to the pelvic organs, which may in turn be affected by hormonal changes and psychological difficulties

MEN

- Small tears in the frenulum can be extremely painful. Wearing a condom for a while after the tear has healed helps to prevent it happening again.
- Retraction of a tight foreskin with erection may be painful and may need circumcision
- Infection, particularly that due to herpes, or deformities of the penis can cause pain on intercourse
- Sexual arousal, not relieved by ejaculation, sometimes leads to aching in the scrotum or the groin region

- Small cysts in the epididymus can be tender when compressed, as well as often causing anxiety
- A hydrocoele, or hernias that come into the scrotum, cause mechanical difficulties and discomfort during intercourse

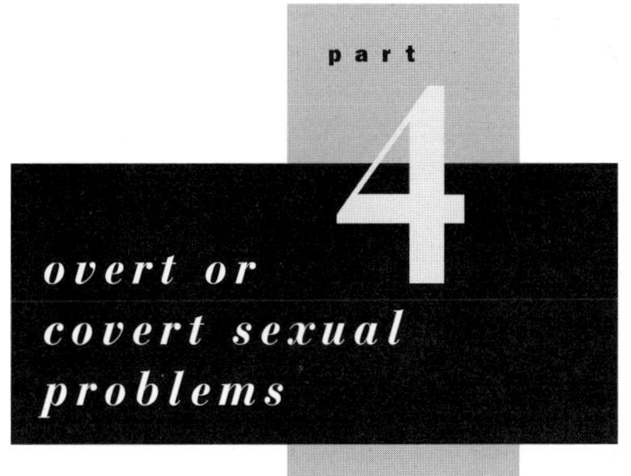

Classification of sexual complaints

WOMEN
- lack of sexual interest in self or partner
- anxiety about sexual matters: gender, masturbation, sexual practices
- non-consummation
- unsatisfactory sex
  - lack of feeling
  - dislike of contact
  - sexual activity tolerated but no arousal
  - arousal but no orgasm
  - clitoral but no vaginal orgasm
  - unsatisfactory orgasm

MEN
- lack of sexual interest in self or partner
- anxiety about sexual matters: gender, masturbation, sexual practices
- lack of erection or too soft for penetration
- poor erection or loss of erection too soon
- ejaculatory too soon
  too late
  none (dry or retrograde)
- dissatisfaction with orgasm

WOMEN/MEN
- sometimes both partners have problems!

Vaginal fantasies

Vaginal fantasies occur frequently.They have to emerge, sometimes at the time of examination, as they are not accessible by direct questioning. Never jump to conclusions about other people's fantasies on the basis of what you have heard from others, or what you might have within yourself. Clever ideas prevent patients explaining or exploring their own fantasies[9].

Many women think of the hymen as a thick barrier, to be broken or torn with much pain and bleeding. The fact that they menstruate, or even have had a baby, has no impact on the fantasy.

Men also have fantasies about the vagina. These may prevent erection, cause loss of erection when approaching the vagina, or prevent ejaculation.

Vaginal fantasies

The entrance
- blocked partially or completely
- hidden
- absent
- within another entrance (cloacal)

The passage
- small or narrow
- blocked
- curved
- absent (has to be made by breaking)
- dangerous, eg with teeth
- disgusting, eg slimy or pus filled

The walls
- rigid – will not stretch
- fragile – will tear
- convoluted – easy to get lost
- raw – like raw meat

The top
- open to the womb
- leads to the inside – to the liver, kidneys or intestines
- enormous cavity – can get lost

Understanding factors in sexual problems following childbirth

Some of the factors in postpartum sexual problems:

- perineal pain – physical/psychological
- fantasies of damage
- actual damage – tears, incontinence, etc
- unresolved feelings about the delivery
    - failure as a woman
    - feelings of exposure
    - feelings of being out of control
    - associating the vagina with pain
- interest/emotion centred on the baby
- jealousy of the baby
- conflict between role of mother and lover
- conflict between breasts as erotic or for breast-feeding
- vaginal dryness due to breast-feeding
- postnatal depression
- fear of further pregnancy
- alteration of partner's view of the woman
- fantasies of the male about the vagina
    - belonging to someone else
    - damaged
    - dangerous
- flashbacks to delivery by either partner

Often patients date their problems to the birth of a baby. Remember that other changes may have been taking place at the same time – moving house, separation or loss of parents, loss of job or status, etc.

Problems may have existed before, but had been tolerated because of the desire for a baby, or an expectation that all would be solved by the birth.

It is important not to assume that the problem is just due to the delivery, and to explore the other areas. It can sometimes be quite difficult to establish a problem arising in the man, because of his peripheral presence in the post-natal environment.

Erectile dysfunction

Most men will experience erectile failure at some time. Across all ages it appears to occur in about 10 per cent of men, increasing in frequency with age[10].

Although it has become apparent that physical causes are common, remember that men will also have *feelings* of inadequacy and loss of manliness with *any* cause. The sexual history will give clues suggestive of the causation – a sudden onset is more likely to indicate a primarily psychological cause.

Treatment includes exploring the psychological problems occurring at the onset and subsequently. Offer physical therapy with injections, vacuum devices or treatment of the underlying cause (where possible).

GENERAL EXAMINATION

- gynaecomastia, palmar erythema, spider naevae, leukonychia
- hypogonadism, loss of secondary sexual characteristics
- thyroid disease
- cardiovascular or peripheral vascular disease
- neurological deficits

INVESTIGATIONS

- full blood count
- liver function tests
- renal function tests
- thyroid function test
- blood sugar
- testosterone
- luteinising hormone
- prolactin

COMMON PHYSICAL CAUSES

- vascular disease
- neurological disease or damage
- diabetes mellitus
- drugs
- peyronies disease
- hormonal deficiency (pituitary, androgen, or other)

Ejaculatory difficulties

Premature or retarded ejaculation can lead to patient and partner dissatisfaction with intercourse. A careful sexual history may reveal unrealistic expectations of simultaneous orgasm or comparisons with erotic fiction.

TREATMENT FOR PREMATURE EJACULATION

- adjustment of the responsibility for success between the couple
- behavioural sensate focus techniques
- squeeze technique
- clomiprimine[11] or a serotonin inhibitor 2-3 hours before intercourse (but beware those with intermittent impotence who will be worse)
- local anaesthetic (lignocaine spray) 5-10 minutes before intercourse[12]

TREATMENT FOR RETARDED EJACULATION

- exploration of the power dynamics in the relationship
- exploration of the feelings of the man about intercourse and the vagina
- treatment of anxiety
- exploration of any fantasies that may be inhibitory
- discontinue drug treatment that may be causative

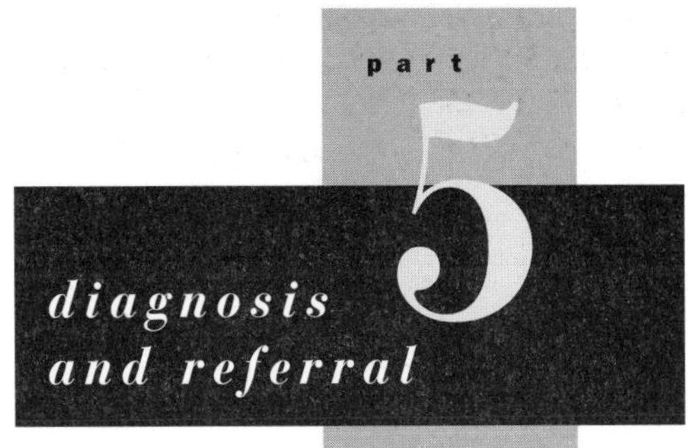

part 5 *diagnosis and referral*

A skilled doctor or nurse can manage most sexual problems in general practice. Postgraduate training for non-specialists is available mainly from courses organised either by the Institute of Psychosexual Medicine[13] or approved by the British Association of Sexual and Marital Therapists[14].

Consider referral if:

- the patient or couple do not want to discuss their problems with someone they know
- the problem is beyond the competence of the doctor or nurse
- the problem requires specialised or lengthy treatment not available in general practice and *the patient wants referral.*

Diagnosis	**Referral facility**
Part of a marital problem	Relate
Part of a psychiatric illness	psychiatrist
Long-standing personality problems or damage, eg survivor of childhood sexual abuse	social worker/ self-help group/ psychologist
Focused psychosexual problem with an otherwise stable personality.	psychosexual clinic
Part of a general inability to cope with relationships	counsellor/ psychologist

Table 1. Common medical problems leading to sexual difficulties

	Problem	Possible solutions
Asthma	Fear of provoking an attack	Use inhaler before intercourse
Arthritis	Pain, weakness, limited movement, tiredness Limitation of external rotation of the hips makes opening the thighs difficult Pelvic thrusting increases back pain	Changes in established sexual positions may enable activity to continue Adequate pain relief before activity
Cardio-vascular	Either partner may have fears of death especially during intercourse. (Rare 0.6% of sudden deaths) Angina Impotence due to arterial damage, treatment, or psychological	Counselling and education about the risks Angina prophylaxis and avoidance of a large meal or excess alcohol beforehand A more active role taken by the healthier partner
Cervical smears and cancer of cervix	Guilt or anger with partner arises from the publicity about links between cervical cancer and early sexual activity, multiple partners or infection After treatment intercourse may be prohibited and this may be interpreted by patients as 'sex is bad', as punishment for sexuality, or as being tainted Inelastic scar tissue may follow treatment Fear of death or contamination of the partner	Counselling and education Avoidance of attitudes of blame Careful choice of words and attitude during examinations and treatments to prevent the development of dysmorphic fantasies
Colostomy or ileostomy	Adjustment to visible passage of urine or faeces Orgasm can cause reflex filling of the bag Pressure on the bag may be uncomfortable Tender scar tissue Damage to nerves causing failure of erection Removal of the rectum is particularly distressing in a homosexual relationship	Changing and taping flat the bag before intercourse Changes in position, eg the 'spoons position', to avoid pressure on the abdomen
Contraception	Fear of pregnancy inhibits sexual desire or response Removal of the risk can reduce excitement Religious or cultural objections can cause guilt If one of a couple uses contraception to please the other, resentment follows Absent periods can be seen as unfeminine Heavy bleeding may be off-putting Fantasies about intrauterine devices may be inhibiting Barrier methods can be a barrier to intimacy Sterilisation or vasectomy can signal the end of sexuality not just fertility	Essential to match the method of contraception to the needs of the couple An excellent method is no good if it is not used because it interferes with sexual function

	Problem	Possible solutions
Diabetes	Reduction in blood supply causes loss of function in genitals or secondary damage to hormone levels Damage to the nervous system causes alteration in sensation and failure of function Impotence occurs in 35-59% of diabetic men, increasing with age Failure of emission may also occur Most women report no problems except those due to local vaginal changes or infections	It is tempting to ascribe sexual difficulties in diabetes to the disease, but they cannot be taken in isolation from the effects of any long-term disability History, investigation and treatment should be available as for any other failure of function
Hysterectomy	Altered sensation if the uterus was enlarged Temporary hormonal loss can occur Scar tissue may be tight Loss of lubrication during healing Loss of fertility may inhibit those couples who think intercourse is only for making babies Some people feel that a woman is not feminine without a uterus The woman, or her partner, may fear the operation has made her too weak to withstand intercourse	Counselling and information Hormone replacement and/or lubricants Removal of the cause of pain, excess bleeding, or discomfort may improve sexual function[15]
Mental handicap	Often regarded as children with no sexuality Often live segregated from others Limited opportunities for appropriate sexual education May be abused or exploited	Sexual needs must be acknowledged Privacy must be available Appropriate sex education essential
Mental illness	Loss of libido common in depression Performance anxiety worsened by panic attacks or anxiety Drug treatment may affect function Manic illness can be accompanied by lack of inhibition, excessive demands, or a belief that they are irresistible	Treatment of the underlying disorder Change of treatment if function affected Sexuality usually returns to pre-morbid condition after recovery
Menopause	Media representations of sex being for the young and vigorous may inhibit activity A view that sex is for reproduction may cause sexual activity to cease Infirmity or death of parents, or loss of mothering role may make this a time of adjustment and change Poor communication and lack of warmth between a couple may have been hidden by the demands of the growing family until now Realisation that the aspirations of the young adult will not be attained may cause a 'mid-life crisis' Menopausal hot sweats, tiredness, etc can reduce desire and cause marital discord Vaginal dryness causes a sore vagina and a sore penis	Hormone replacement therapy may solve the woman's problems, leaving the man confronted by an increasingly inadequate erection A couple with sexual problems at the menopause should examine the causes just as they would at any other age, not expect hormone replacement therapy to cure them all

Table 1. Common medical problems leading to sexual difficulties (continued)

	Problem	Possible solutions
Menopause *contd*	The man may become afraid of hurting his partner Anxiety about pain reduces lubrication, and may affect the erection The fall in hormone levels with reduced blood supply leads to loss of elasticity and sensation	
Prescribed medication	Drugs are used to treat medical condition which may themselves be the cause of sexual problems Psychological reactions to illness, or the need to take drug treatment may affect sexuality	Always ask open ended questions like 'How's the love life?' or 'Have you noticed any difference in your sex life?'
Prolapse	Mechanical obstruction to penis within the vagina Forcible movement of prolapsed tissues during intercourse causes discomfort or pain Bladder or rectum may empty	If allowed to persist, avoidance of intercourse is common Alteration of positions after repair may be necessary because of tender scar tissue
Prostate enlargement	Finasteride treatment may cause impotence Trans-urethral surgery rarely causes impotence Retrograde ejaculation after surgery is common	Counselling and information Alternative medical treatments such as alpha-blockers
Recreational drugs (including alcohol)	Difficult to separate the expectations from the effects Erectile problems are common Orgasm and ejaculation usually delayed The high of a fix may be substituted for orgasm Loss of inhibition may lead to risky sexual practices	Address the psychological and interpersonal difficulties underlying the addictive behaviour Advise condom use
Spinal injuries	Sexual desire is not usually affected once the immediate effects are over Bowel or bladder dysfunction increases psychological problems Spastic muscles cause problems with some positions Orgasm may be altered, absent, or just as before, despite little or no sensation in the genital area Many will have a normal erection, but not all ejaculate High spinal cord damage can cause a distressing condition in which sexual stimulation triggers headache, flushing and sweating	Most people with spinal cord damage return to satisfying sexual activity despite considerable nerve damage Pain and lack of mobility require alterations in technique and positions The non-affected partner may need to become more active
Strokes	Sexual desire usually seems to return to normal after 6-7 weeks unless psychological fears interfere Occasionally understanding of when sexual activity is appropriate is altered and may cause offence Physical disabilities require alterations as above There is no evidence for the common fear that another stroke may be caused by sexual activity	Counselling and education Willingness to alter established patterns of positions, activity, etc makes resumption of sexual activity more likely

	Problem	Possible solutions
Sexually transmitted infections (STIs)	Discomfort and pain inhibit desire and response The stigma associated with infections can upset the relationship, especially if an outside liaison is suspected The feelings about the genitals, or about possible infidelity, can last long after the original infection	Counselling and information A non-judgmental attitude is essential Acceptance of other people's sexual behaviour is important, while pointing out the dangers if necessary
Phobias about STIs	The anxiety may have its basis in the prohibition of sexual thoughts or actions in childhood, or by religion Sufferers attend repeatedly for testing and are not reassured by a negative result Sufferers may avoid intimacy with their partners, fearing they will infect them	Exploration of the inner fears and sexual prohibitions Avoid repeated testing

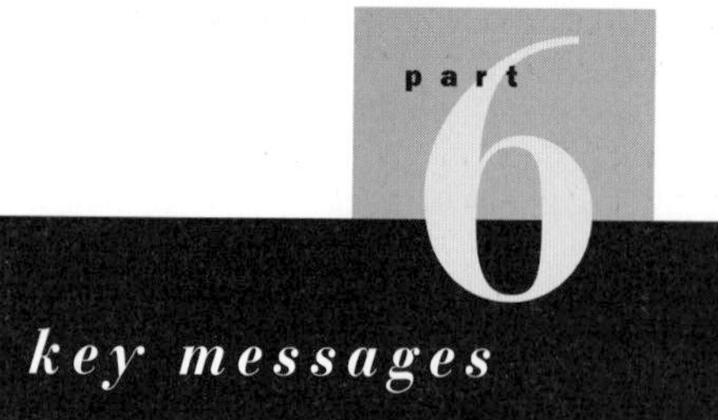

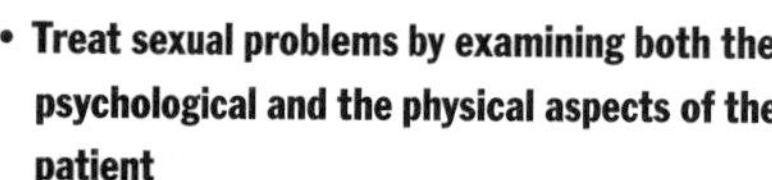

part 6 key messages

- Treat sexual problems by examining both the psychological and the physical aspects of the patient
- Include a sexual history in your consultations unless it is obviously not required
- Most patients will tell you the nature of the problem if you allow them to do so using open-ended questions
- Health professionals do not need to be expert at sexual therapy to obtain an adequate sexual history
- Many patients can be helped to resolve their problems in short consultations
- Give reassurance only after you and the patient both understand the nature of the problem
- Improve your own skills in the interpretation of the doctor-patient relationship to help those with simple problems
- Limit offers of help to those who want to work to change
- Know where you can refer those patients beyond your level of expertise or who request referral

part 7 further reading

- ***Contraceptive care: meeting individual needs***
  Montford H and Skrine R
  Chapman & Hall, 1993

- ***Introduction to psychosexual medicine***
  Skrine R
  Chapman & Hall, 1989

- ***Insights into troubled sexuality***
  Tunnadine P
  Chapman & Hall, 1992

- ***Sexual health promotion in general practice***
  Curtis H, Hoolaghan T and Jewitt C
  Radcliffe Medical Press, 1995

- ***Human sexuality and its problems***
  Bancroft J
  Churchill Livingstone, 1989

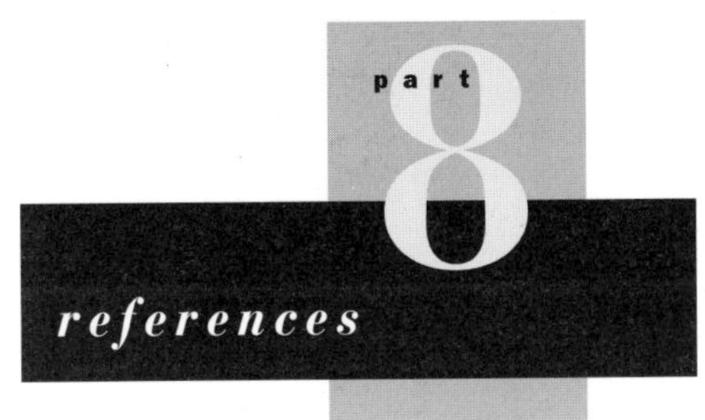

part 8 references

1 'Sexual dysfunction among middle aged women in the community', Osborne M, ***British Medical Journal, 296,*** 1988, 959-962

2 ***The impact of sexual problems in the general population: dissertation for the Diploma in Epidemiology,*** Dunn KM, Keele University, 1996

3 ***Contraceptive care: meeting individual needs,*** Montford H and Skrine R, (eds), Chapman & Hall, 1993

4 ***Discussing sexuality: a guide for health professionals,*** Ross MW and Channon-Little LD, MacLennan and Petty, Sydney, 1991

5 ***The doctor, his patient and the illness,*** Balint M, Pitman, 1964

6 ***The inner consultation,*** Neighbour R, Petroc Press, 1987.

7 ***Human sexuality and its problems,*** Bancroft J, Churchill Livingstone, 1989

8 ***Blocks and freedoms in sexual life,*** Skrine R, Radcliffe Medical Press, 1997

9 ***Vaginismus: understanding and overcoming the blocks to intercourse,*** Valins L, Ashgrove Press, 1988

10 'Frequency of sexual dysfunction in 'normal' couples', Frank E, Anderson C and Rubenstein D, ***New England Journal of Medicine, 299,*** 1987, 111-15

11 'Clomiprimine versus placebo in the treatment of premature ejaculation: a pilot study', Segraves RT, Saren A, Segraves K, Maguire E, ***Journal of Sexual and Marital Therapy, 19,*** 1993, 198-200

12 'Premature Ejaculation', Riley A, ***Journal of Sexual Health, 4,*** 1994, 69-71

13 Institute of Psychosexual Medicine, 11 Chandos Street, London W1M 9DE

14 British Association of Sexual and Marital Therapy, PO Box 62, Sheffield S10 3TS

15 'Women's subjective experience of hysterectomy' Ferroni P and Deeble J, ***Australian Health Review, 19,*** 1996, 40-55

Louis Levy

Theresa Nash

11

chapter eleven

building primary care teams for sexual health

part

I

introduction

It is widely recognised that effective team work within primary care leads to staff and patient benefits[1-3]. However, there has been great debate about the *functioning* of primary care teams. We also know that, in practice, team building can be problematic especially where there are communication breakdowns, interpersonal conflicts and leadership issues[4-6].

In order to work successfully with patients on emotive subjects such as sex, sexuality and sexual health, a creative, flexible and innovative approach to working is often required. The need for an effective supportive team is essential to achieve this. This chapter considers how to promote general practice team work, suggests roles for primary care team members, looks at the support structures that may be required and at outcomes in terms of sexual health service development.

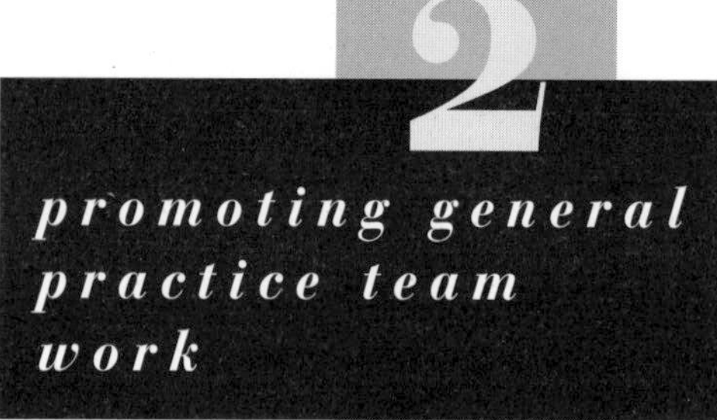

promoting general practice team work

Any well-functioning general practice team is likely to possess the following qualities[4,7].

- a common goal or vision for the team
- respect and understanding of members' variant skills and knowledge, including the uniqueness of their role
- support and development for individual roles
- the ability to listen, both to team members and to patients' views and concerns
- acceptance and management of conflict

There are often numerous ways of responding to an issue. Members need to work towards unity by acknowledging differences of opinion and questioning them in a positive way. In order to achieve these qualities, teams need to consider the following key factors which have been suggested as leading to innovative practice[8].

- *Vision and shared objectives:* does the team have clearly defined objectives? Are these shared by all members? This is essential if teams are to have focus and direction
- *Facilitating participation:* is information shared within the team? Are there regular team meetings? Do all members feel they have input into the decision making process? Do team members experience the team as supportive, co-operative and interpersonally non-threatening?
- *Support for innovation:* Are team members encouraged to develop new ways of working?

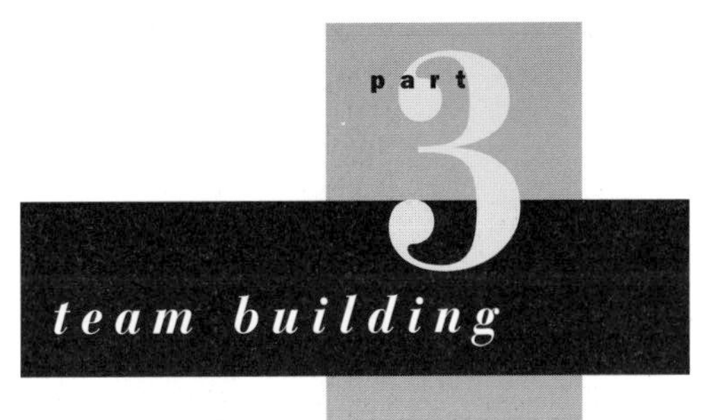

Team leadership

Often the GP is seen as the team leader as they are seen to carry the ultimate responsibility for patient care. However *shared leadership* and delegation of responsibilities has been shown to be more effective[5]. Developing a democratic leadership style involves encouraging full discussion, freedom of working methods and objective praise and criticism. Democratic styles create more effective team working than autocratic or laissez-faire leadership[7].

As with other areas of work identifying who will lead service developments is essential to keep sexual health service provision on the primary health care team (PHCT) agenda.

Phases of team development

Tuckman[9] suggested four distinct phases through which group members have to pass before they become an effective team:

- *forming:* team members meet and begin to formulate their purpose, objectives and goals
- *storming:* identifying group skills, developing standards of behaviour, allocating areas of responsibility and individual roles. Conflicts inevitably arise and need to be resolved to the mutual satisfaction of all before movement to the next stage
- *norming:* acceptance of shared group norms. A group norm is described as a common viewpoint or standard to which all members are expected to subscribe
- *performing:* objectives are achieved through a stable pattern of personal relationships and roles are mutually understood and agreed

Teams are often at different stages of development. It is important to acknowledge this but also to identify further support in the development process. During all stages the use of an outside facilitator can be particularly helpful in developing the team, providing support and passing on skills to team leaders[10-12].

Establishing a team

In order to achieve 'functional' working particularly, when developing sexual health services the primary care team needs defining. Primary care teams are individualistic serving a unique population, but all practices will have a core team.

It is essential to consider who provides sexual health services to the practice population in order to:

- ensure a team approach to future developments, to ensure ownership of policies, guidelines and audit
- facilitate the sharing of knowledge and experience to identify staff training needs and to consider how best to meet these
- ensure staff receive support, especially when responding to emotive situations
- develop liaison with other service providers and ensure referral procedures are clear, this can be useful to gain advice on approaches for example when responding to the needs of black and ethnic minority groups or working with people with learning disabilities
- consider new ways of advertising service provision

The core team includes: receptionists, practice nurses, nurse practitioners, practice managers, health visitors, general practitioners and district nurses.

The wider team, with whom members of the core team work, or liaise with, includes: community midwives, counsellors, community psychiatric nurses, nurse specialists, school nurses, community outreach workers and youth workers.

LOCAL SERVICE PROVIDERS

Both the core team and wider team members may need to liaise with other sexual health service providers. Knowledge of these referral routes is essential. These service providers include: family planning clinics, young persons clinics, termination services, psychosexual counselling, GUM services, substance use projects, lesbian, gay and bisexual community groups, black and ethnic minority groups, outreach workers, natural fertility teachers, rape crisis centres, Relate and the local health promotion department.

Core team meetings
While team meetings cannot guarantee better team working they are fundamental to the process of collaborative working. Managing meetings requires an understanding of the internal team processes[13]. Firth-Cozens[7] quotes Anthony Jay's guide to leading meetings:

- control the garrulous
- draw out the silent
- protect the weak
- encourage the clash of ideas
- watch out for the suggestion squashing reflex
- come to the most senior people last
- close on a note of achievement

Practices may wish to consider the advantages of facilitated meetings, which have been shown to enable all team members to contribute and to feel ownership of future developments.

The use of facilitators to work with PHCTs in developing sexual history taking guidelines is most successful if a 'bottom up' approach is used:

- it ensures team ownership by building upon existing skills, knowledge and experience
- it reflects the variability of practice resources and cultures
- it enables greater flexibility in the way developed guidelines are used[14]

Roles and responsibilities
Key considerations in the development of team members' roles are:

- individual skills, knowledge and motivation
- the recognition of role overlaps
- members being aware of their own values and attitudes to sex, sexuality and the provision of sexual health services
- members being aware of confidentiality issues as it pertains to their role
- members being able to recognise and articulate their needs for further training

Some suggestions for core team members' roles in providing sexual health services are included opposite.

Practice manager

- ongoing support for team members including encouragement to attend courses
- co-ordination of meetings/projects and ensuring dissemination of information
- audit role

Receptionist

- 'face of the service', as first point of contact important in reassuring patients
- need to be aware of all team members' roles in order to ensure referrals to appropriate practitioner when responding to patient queries
- aware of emergency contraception time limits and referral points, including outside agencies
- fully involved in team meetings

Practice nurse/nurse practitioner

- dependent on skills involved in all aspects of sexual health service provision, eg well man and well woman screening, contraception, travel, cervical smear, emergency contraception, ante-natal, postnatal (clear overlap with GP's role)
- opportunistic sexual health history taking
- discussing confidentiality with clients
- resource within practice for health education materials, internal and external referral routes, eg counselling services
- often recognised by patients as having more time to discuss concerns

The practice nurse role has been shown to be under-utilised in the provision of sexual health services[15].

General practitioner

- supporting and acknowledging role of team members, valuing training and team meetings
- maintaining confidentiality including written records and reports, eg insurance and employer reports (see Chapter 3, page 58).
- sexual health history taking during variant consultations, eg fertility, psychosexual, mental health, substance use, review of diabetes, beta blockers (link to impotence), recurrent visits for non specific symptoms, contraception, termination referrals, vaginal discharge
- being aware of referral routes both internal and external to practice

Health visitor

- raising awareness of sexual health issues both with individual patients, their families and within community work as appropriate
- opportunistic sexual history taking during ante-natal and postnatal visits

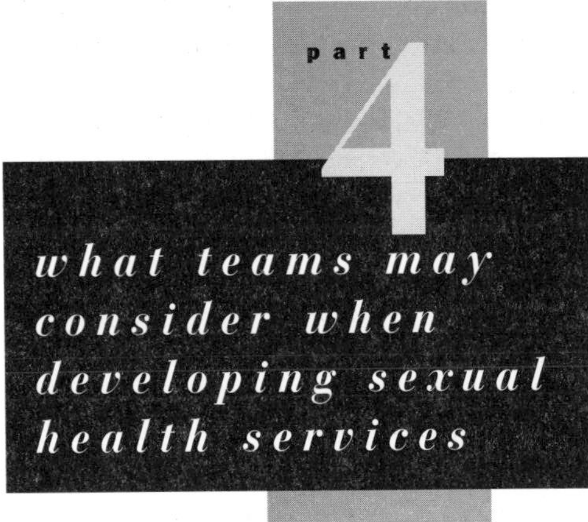

(See also see Chapter 12.)

See Table 1, page 167.

Setting objectives

Following the sexual health service audit clear objectives can be defined. These need to be specific, measurable, achievable, realistic and timed, that is SMART. This method of developing objectives can be used to prioritise first 'action' points.

EXAMPLE

Smart for condoms!

Specific
To provide free condoms to sexually active patients/clients particularly those who may be practising high risk activities

Measurable
Monitor number and type of condoms distributed and document safer sex discussion

Achievable
If have access to resources and have the skills to discuss sex and safer sex

Realistic
Information collected on present computer fields for safe sex advice and condom use. Monitor distribution as a stock control procedure (not per individual consultation)

Timed
Review with staff quarterly (set review date)
Collate monitoring criteria for one month each quarter

Monitoring team work
Once the objective(s) are agreed, consider training needs, guidelines development, implementation process, who else needs to be involved and the review date.

Joint ownership
As previously discussed it is important that the whole team takes part in the discussions when developing sexual health services. Different staff members will have different views on how to achieve objectives.

case study

A condom project was introduced in a practice where the receptionists had not been involved in the team training or discussions, even though they were to be involved in the distribution. It was discovered that when young people asked for condoms they were only given one if the receptionists thought they looked under eighteen. It transpired that the receptionists were unclear about the law as it relates to young people and were very uncomfortable about distributing condoms.

If they had been fully involved in the planning stage of this development their fears could have been discussed and any training needs met.

Research has shown that many doctors and nurses have reservations about working with certain types of patients, due to sex, age and cultural differences[15]. This can create a barrier when offering services in that sexual health issues are avoided. Unless time is given to explore professionals' fears and mechanisms introduced to overcome them, then certain clients will not have access to sexual health services.

Some male doctors feel very uncomfortable raising sexual health issues with young female patients, due to fear of this being misread by patients. This could be overcome by agreeing that referrals are made to the practice nurse and stating this clearly to the patient.

SOCIAL NETWORKS
Where health professionals provide services to friends, colleagues, neighbours or acquaintances, raising sexual health can be embarrassing. This needs to be acknowledged and appropriate referral routes considered.

Added value
A team approach to developing sexual health service provision has been shown to have positive outcomes in the 'knock on' effect for other initiatives, for instance in developing asthma and diabetic clinics.

Table 1: Review/audit current sexual health service provision

Data collection may include:	Suggested area for inclusion
Demographic data:	Total practice population, age/sex breakdown, description of ethnic minority groups, conception rate by maternal age and outcome of pregnancy, uptake of emergency contraception
Present contraceptive provision and uptake	Is information available on all methods? Is information given advising patients where they can access methods not available at the practice?
Resource availability	Staff skills and knowledge • consider the gender mix of the core team • consider the need to be sensitive to the composition of the practice population Literature • are leaflets available in relevant languages? • is literature available on alternative service providers? • is there a named person to co-ordinate resource ordering and display, eg ensuring leaflet stocks are up to date? • are leaflets being regularly given out, eg the FPA's Contraceptive Education Service method leaflets?
Advertising of services	• is the availability of emergency contraception publicised in your practice? • is information on sexual health and contraception services included in your practice leaflet?
Current sexual health guidelines	eg confidentiality, sexual history taking, responding to HIV test requests, condom distribution, emergency contraception provision.
Training and support needs of staff	recognising the need for further training can be incorporated into facilitated meetings, as staff may need support in identifying those areas they find uncomfortable responding to

part 5

key messages

- Recognising the importance of team development for the effective delivery of sexual health services is essential
- Confidentiality and issues relating to team members' attitudes need addressing initially as these are fundamental to the development of accessible services. They also underpin guideline development, eg for sexual history taking, HIV testing and condom distribution (agreement about the recording of information is essential)
- The process of service development can seem overwhelming. Start small with manageable initiatives, eg advertising emergency contraception provision, ensuring literature available in a variety of languages, developing a list of local service providers, ensuring receptionists are aware of time limits for emergency contraception

further reading and support

- ***Sexual history taking in general practice***
  Jewitt C
  The HIV Project, 1995

- ***Team development: a manual of facilitation for health educators and promoters***
  Rolls L
  Health Education Authority, 1992

- ***Practice makes perfect: a sexual health resource for primary care***
  Whetton T
  Bexley & Greenwich Health 1996 (available from Durex Information Service)

- ***Discussing sex: a guide to good practice for sexual health promotion and HIV prevention for primary care settings***
  Levy LB
  The HIV Project, 1997

The following organisations have experience in facilitating sexual health services with primary care teams:

The HIV Project
St Martins House
3rd Floor
140 Tottenham Court Road
London
W1 P 9LN
tel 0171 383 0770

Oasis Humans Relations
The Centre for Development Education
Hall Mews, Clifford Road
Boston Spa
Wetherby, West Yorks
LS23 6DT
tel 01937 541700

part 7

references

1 ***Quality in General Practice: Policy statement (2),*** Royal College of General Practitioners, 1985

2 ***Interprofession collaboration in primary health care organisations***, Gregson B, Cartlidge A and Bono J, Occasional Paper 52, Royal College of General Practitioners, 1991

3 'The primary care team', Waine C, ***British Journal of General Practice, 42***, 1992, 498–99

4 'Paths to effective teamwork in primary care settings', Cook R, ***Nursing Times, 92***, 1996, 44–45

5 'Primary health care team workshop: team members' perspectives', Long S, ***Journal of Advanced Nursing, 23***, 1996, 935–41

6 'Teamwork in primary care: the views and experiences of nurses, midwives and health visitors', Wiles R, ***Journal of Advanced Nursing, 20***, 1994, 324–30

7 'Building teams for effective audit', Firth-Cozens J, ***Quality in Health Care, 1***, 1992, 252–55

8 'Effective multidisciplinary teamwork in primary health care', Poulton B and West M, ***Journal of Advanced Nursing, 18***, 1993, 918–25

9 'Team playing', Eggert M, ***Nursing Standard, 8 (28), 1994,*** 49–54

10 'The facilitation of multiprofessional clinical audit in primary health care teams – from audit to quality assurance', Baker R, Sorrie R, Reddish S, et al, ***Journal of Interprofessional Care 9(3), 1995***, 237–44

11 'Educational potential of medical audit: observations from a study of small groups setting standards', Newton J, Hutchinson A and Steen N, et al, ***Quality in Health Care, 1, 1992,*** 256–59

12 'Multidisciplinary audit in primary healthcare teams: facilitation by audit support staff', Hearnshaw H, Baker R and Robertson N, ***Quality in Health Care, 3***, 1994, 164–68

13 'Promoting collaboration in the primary care team – the role of the practice meeting', Bennett-Emslie G and McIntosh J, ***Journal of Interprofessional Care, 9***, 1995, 251–56

14 ***Sexual history taking in general practice***, Jewitt C,The HIV Project, 1995

15 ***Sexual health and family planning services in general practice. Report of a qualitative research survey in England and Wales***, Institute of Population Studies for the Family Planning Association and Health Education Authority, FPA, 1993

Janet Harris

Andrea Jones

12

chapter twelve

ensuring the quality of sexual health services in primary care

part I introduction

This chapter is designed to provide practical guidance on ways to compare your existing practice with the examples of good practice that are given in this book. For those who wish to obtain more information about assessing clinical care, a suggested reading list can be found at the end of the chapter.

You can review a number of clinical areas from every chapter in this book through critical incident analysis, needs assessment, clinical audit, or service evaluation. This chapter will help you to:

- decide when to review services
- use practice data and comparative data
- choose a method for review
- conduct the review
- implement the results

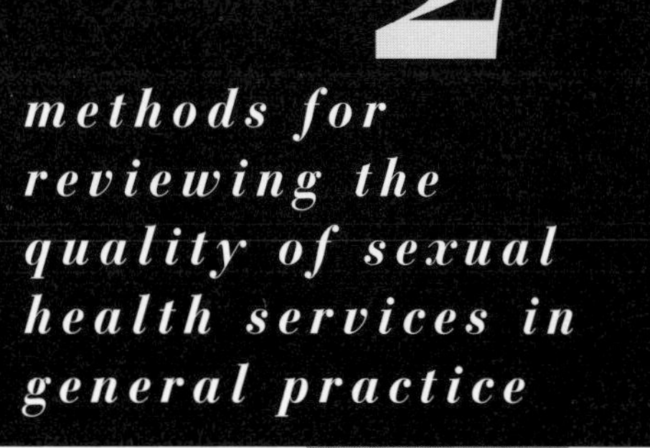

part 2 methods for reviewing the quality of sexual health services in general practice

Critical incident analysis

Critical incident analysis involves members of the primary health care team (PHCT) in examining the factors surrounding an episode of patient care. The incident may have been unusually negative or positive. Analysing a negative incident helps the team to decide whether it is an isolated occurrence, as well as identifying aspects of care which should be changed to prevent the incident from occurring again in the future. Analysing a positive incident can identify aspects of care that can be used by other members of the PHCT with other patients in the future. Examples of significant events might be the occurrence of a blood clot in a patient taking the oral contraceptive pill, a late termination of pregnancy, and infertility due to undetected chlamydia.

Critical incident analysis will involve some or all of the following:

- identification of critical incident
- facilitatation of group discussion amongst all relevant members of PHCT to explore:
  - causative factors
  - courses of action which might prevent recurrence of the incident
  - variations in the clinical practice of members of the PHCT in relation to the incident
- reviewing patient case notes to establish the care given
- reviewing relevant literature to identify

guidelines or evidence to shape future practice
- development of a practice policy

Needs assessment

Responsiveness to local needs is essential when providing sexual health services. Identifying the sexual health needs of the practice population will enable the practice to tailor its services to meet those needs. General practices can use four approaches to needs assessment[1]:

- The ***practice-defined approach:*** which involves the analysis of practice population data. This approach yields useful baseline information on the needs of the patients who use practice services.

- The ***comparative approach:*** which compares practice and community data with data from other general practices, or with district or national level data. This kind of analysis identifies the unique needs of the practice population in comparison with other local and national populations.

- The ***epidemiological approach:*** which defines need in terms of the incidence and prevalence of disease. This approach can include a review of the services available in relation to a particular condition and the way in which such services are used. It also attempts to determine the clinical and cost effectiveness of the services currently provided.

- The ***patient-defined approach:*** which involves people in defining needs and priorities from the patients' point of view. This approach obtains useful information from patients who may not use practice services regularly, or who do not routinely express their needs.

Clinical audit is:

*'the systematic and critical analysis of the quality of clinical care, including the procedures used for diagnosis, treatment and care, the associated use of resources and the resulting outcome and quality of life for the patient' (*NHS Executive, 1996[2])

Clinical audit enables a service to compare its current practice with relevant evidence-based standards and to identify changes required to bring the service in line. The clinical audit cycle consists of six main stages which should all be completed in order for the audit to be effective. The audit cycle is shown below.

Standards for audit should be based on research evidence of clinical effectiveness where it is available. Evidence is graded on its strength in the following order:

1 Randomised controlled trials

2 Other robust experimental or observations studies

3 Structured consensus of experts in the field

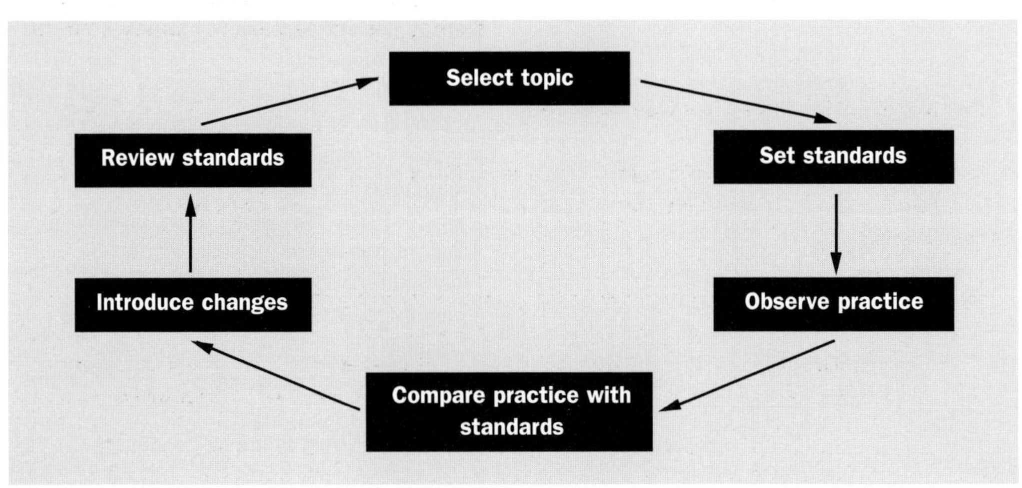

Where evidence of clinical effectiveness is not available, standards for practice audit should be based on one of the following:

- patient views/needs
- consensus of relevant PHCT members
- legislation

Service evaluation

Service evaluations are conducted to:

- determine the degree of attainment of service objectives
- identify the strengths and weaknesses of a service
- improve the professional's skill in the performance of evaluation activities
- fulfil grant or contract requirements
- determine whether a service can be used in other populations/settings
- contribute to the base of knowledge about sexual health service design[3].

Evaluations can use some of the methods that are used in critical incident analysis, clinical audit and needs assessment. They are most commonly used to review the impact of new services or changes in service delivery across clinical settings and districts. Results are used to inform health care policy, make decisions about large scale modifications to service structure and delivery, and to build an evidence base for best practice. General practices may participate in a service evaluation that is commissioned by a locality or commissioning authority, but it is unlikely that a single practice would have reason to co-ordinate a service evaluation.

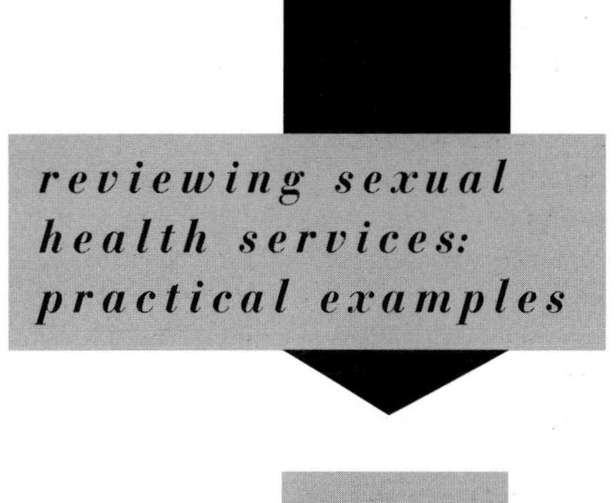

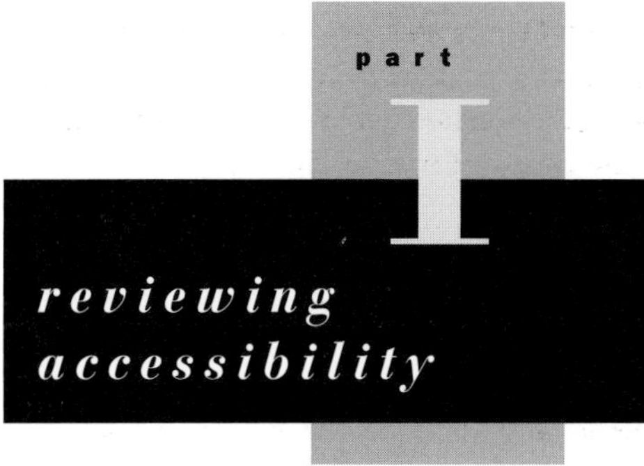

example

A patient requests emergency contraception but is too late for it to be prescribed

Patient review of critical incident

Ask the patient to draw a line on a sheet of paper. At the beginning of the line, ask them to put a mark where they first thought of needing emergency contraception. Then ask them to list out each event that occurred from

Patient experiences of barriers to access

- needed emergency contraception
- called practice
- had to tell them what I wanted
- hung up
- got a friend to call
- they wanted me to come in during school
- I probably don't need it anyway
- here today for a pregnancy test

when they first thought of calling the practice. An analysis of this incident would involve patients and members of the PHCT in:

- discussing the barriers to accessing services
- identifying strategies for removing barriers, which might prevent it happening again in the future
- reviewing the situation with other patients who request the service, to establish whether procedures should be changed in the future to prevent such an occurrence

Some possible solutions are:

- training receptionists about scheduling confidential emergency appointments
- publicising ways to access emergency contraception[4]. For example, Schering produce a 'priority appointment request card' which women can give to the receptionist instead of having to discuss their need for an emergency contraception appointment.

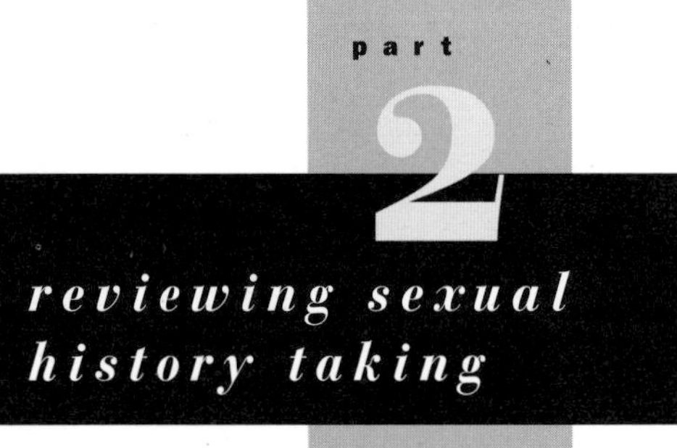

STAFF REVIEW OF CRITICAL INCIDENTS

Each member of the PHCT brings two examples of sexual history taking to the team meeting – a case where problems were encountered with the history taking, and a case where the history taking went well for both staff and the patient. These are sketched out by drawing the situation in the centre of the page, and listing out the problems and successful factors for each situation: (see diagram opposite).

This exercise gives team members an opportunity to learn successful approaches and strategies from each other, while realising that everyone finds history taking a challenge at one time or another. If the same themes are identified across a number of cases, the team can discuss the need for team training.

Sexual history taking: sketching out problems and success

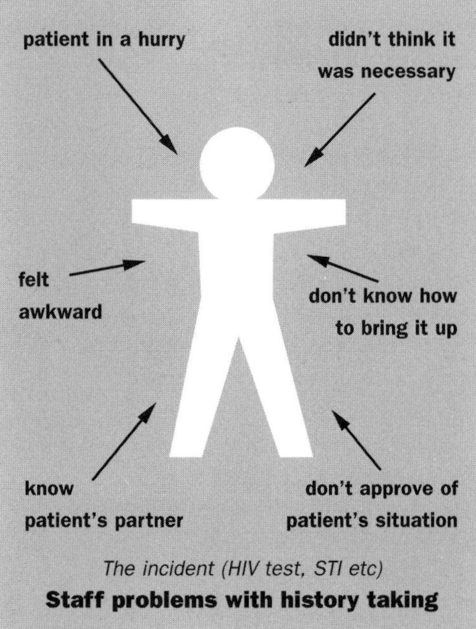

The incident (HIV test, STI etc)

Staff problems with history taking

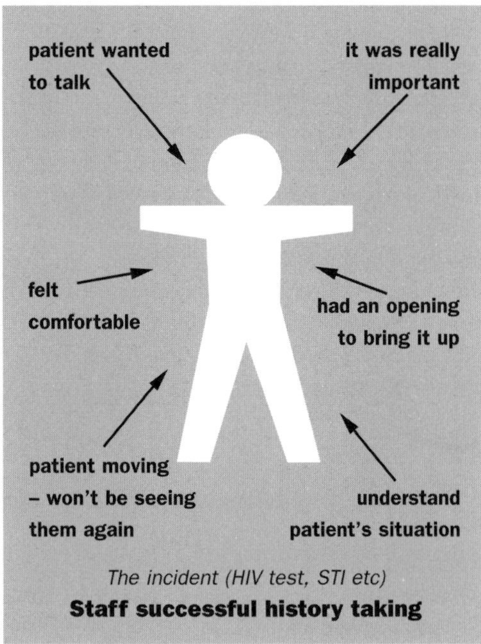

The incident (HIV test, STI etc)

Staff successful history taking

PATIENT REVIEW OF CRITICAL INCIDENTS

The same exercise can be used with patients to identify their concerns and needs regarding sexual history taking. Patients can be asked to think back to positive and negative incidents when they had to talk to a member of the PHCT: (see below).

If patients are consistently mentioning similar problems, then the PHCT might want to consider staff training and/or techniques for helping patients to realise that sexual health discussions are part of routine primary care.

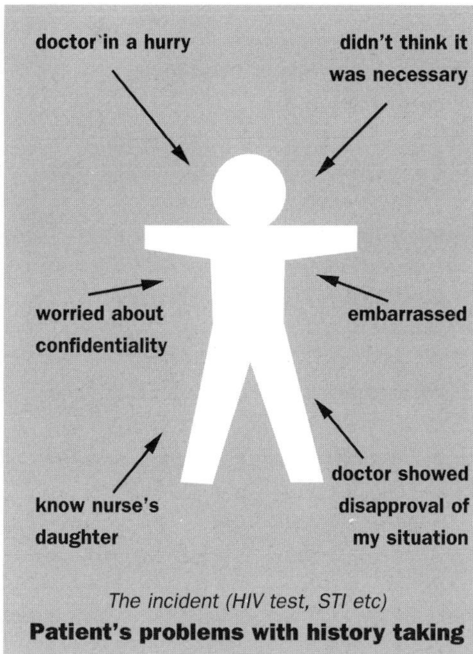

The incident (HIV test, STI etc)

Patient's problems with history taking

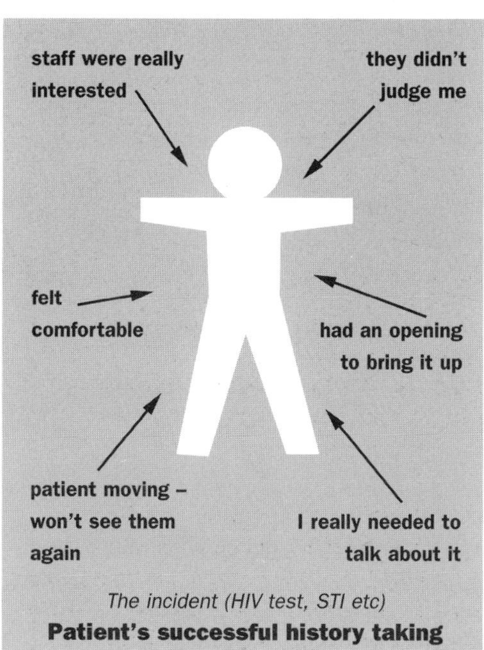

The incident (HIV test, STI etc)

Patient's successful history taking

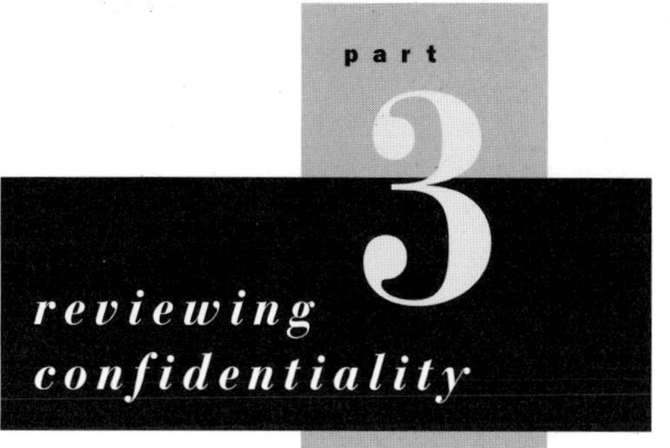

Record security and confidentiality: audit checklist

If your practice answers 'yes' to any of these questions, then you have problems with record security and confidentiality.

- Is there public access to rooms where notes are stored?
- Are notes left in treatment rooms where other patients can see them?
- Are notes easily accessible when out visiting?
- Are computers easily removed from the surgery?
- Do you have passwords that are easy to guess?
- Are faxes sent to receiving machines that are not secure?
- Are redundant paper records left unshredded?
- Does the receptionist ask people to state the reasons for their visit?
- Are reasons for patients' visits kept on a list at the reception desk that can be seen by patients when they check in?
- Can patients overhear the receptionist making appointments?
- Do patients who are being seen for contraception sit in a designated area of the waiting room?
- Do staff who specialise in sexual health call patients in by name?
- Do staff ask relatives (or others with no 'need to know') to translate for patients?
- Do staff assume that they can decide how test results will be communicated without asking the patient?

Discuss how the organisation and layout of the practice can be changed to protect confidentiality.

Staff map of confidentiality within the practice

Have the PHCT work together to draw a rough map of the practice. Use the security and confidentiality checklist shown on previous page to mark areas where there may be problems.

Team assessment of a critical incident

example

A 15 year old girl reports a breach of confidentiality regarding her contraceptive use.

An analysis of this incident would involve relevant members of the PHCT in:

- discussing the factors which might have been involved in causing the event
- identifying courses of action which might prevent it happening again in the future
- reviewing variations in practice with regard to the maintenance of confidentiality, especially with regard to patients who are under 16
- reviewing the patient's case notes to establish whether the care given should or could be changed in the future to prevent such an occurrence
- seeking out guidance on the rights of under 16s and reporting this back to the group· developing a practice policy or a simple checklist to guide practice in the future

Assessing concerns and beliefs about confidentiality

Concerns and beliefs can be identified through a simple survey:

PRACTICE SURVEY ON CONFIDENTIALITY

1 What sort of information should be kept confidential – just between you and your doctor?

---

2 What sort of information could be shared with other members of the practice team?

---

3 Do you have any worries about confidentiality?

---

4 For parents of teenagers: Do you think that you should be told about everything that happens between your son or daughter and your GP? Are there things that should remain confidential?

---

5 For teenagers: Do you think that your parents will be told about your visits to the practice? Are you ever reluctant to visit the practice because your parents might find out?

This can be a written survey that is distributed to parents, or a list of informal questions that all practice staff agree to ask patients across a period of one or two weeks. The results can be used by the team to:

- discuss whether patients' attitudes concur with the PHCT's views of good practice
- put a statement about confidentiality in practice leaflets
- put information about confidentiality on posters in the waiting room

Auditing practice team beliefs about record keeping

The practice team can review their beliefs about what needs to be recorded in the notes, as follows:

1 Bring packets of yellow post-it notes and pens to the meeting.
2 Ask each person in the practice team to write things that should be recorded in the patient's record on post-it notes. Stick all the post-it notes on a section of the wall.

3 Ask team members to write things that should *not* be recorded in the patient's record on post-it notes. Put these notes on a different section of the wall.
4 Ask everyone to look at the notes and identify areas where there is agreement/ disagreement.
5 If the informal review shows that practice staff have different beliefs about record keeping, then the team can discuss why some members feel that the information needs to be recorded. This can be done by reviewing the reasons why information is kept in notes, and the 'worst that could happen' if information is kept in notes.

This exercise can be used to seek out guidance on record keeping and develop a practice policy or a simple checklist to guide practice in the future.

After developing a policy or checklist, the practice can periodically review a sample of patient records to see if there are still variations in record keeping amongst members of the PHCT.

Information that should not be contained in patient records	**Contained in Record Number**							
	1	**2**	**3**	**4**	**5**	**6**	**7**	**8**
Sexual orientation								
Transsexualism								
Names of sexual partners								
Asymptomatic HIV status								
A previous abortion								
Child conceived by donor insemination								
Attendance at a GUM clinic								
Other								

Confidentiality and record keeping pro forma

Investigating current practice regarding disclosure of information

THE TEAM CAN ASK THEMSELVES THE FOLLOWING

Do members of our primary health care team:

- check with the patient before sharing information within the primary health care team?
- confirm the patient's identity before revealing test results or other information?
- obtain the patient's consent before revealing information to others?
- check with the patient before responding to lawyers letters or insurance forms?
- check with the patient/patient's family before giving information on lifestyle and risk of death or disease to external agencies?
- have practice policies on disclosing sexual abuse? Informing partners about HIV infection?
- have practice policies on disclosing information after the patient's death?

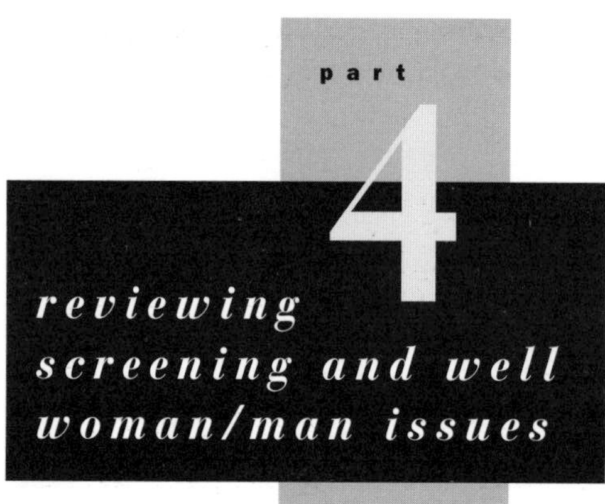

Critical incident analysis in cervical screening

example

A 40 year old woman has been diagnosed with cervical cancer. She has never received a smear.

A critical incident analysis would involve patients and members of the PHCT in:

- looking at the patient's notes to see if she was ever informed of the need for screening
- reviewing practice initiatives for promoting patient awareness about the need for routine screening
- reviewing protocols for contacting patients about cervical screening
- discussing the barriers to accessing cervical screening services with patients
- identifying strategies for removing barriers, which might prevent it happening again in the future
- reviewing protocols that have been used by other practices to promote awareness and increase uptake of screening
- adopting a practice protocol for notifying patients about the need for cervical screening

Assessing cervical screening activity

The critical incident could be viewed within a broader epidemiological context of reviewing the amount of routine screening done within the practice. Screening activity can be determined by:

1 Reviewing the practice register to determine the number of women in the target population – women aged 20-64 years
2 Selecting a random sample (10-20%) of patient records for women who have been on the practice list for the past five years
3 Counting the number of women contacted for cervical screening in the past five years
4 Counting the number of women attending for cervical screening
5 Counting the number of women who were notified of results
6 Calculating the proportion of 20–64 year old women contacted for screening:

$$\frac{\text{Number of women aged 20-64 contacted for screening}}{\text{Number of women aged 20-64 on practice list}} = \text{proportion contacted}$$

7 Calculating the proportion screened of those contacted:

$$\frac{\text{Number of women aged 20-64 attending for screening}}{\text{Number of women aged 20-64 contacted for screening}} = \text{proportion screened}$$

Clinical audit of cervical screening

The epidemiological data shown above can be used to establish standards and targets for screening. Once standards and targets have been set, they can be audited annually to determine the success of the screening programme and to identify variations in practice.

Critical incident analysis in chlamydia screening

example

A 25 year old woman has confirmed infertility due to undetected chlamydia. Over the past year, she has presented to the general practice on three occasions with chronic pelvic pain.

An analysis of this incident would involve members of the PHCT in:

- reviewing the patient's notes to determine clinical signs and reported symptoms
- reviewing staff knowledge of indications for chlamydia screening
- obtaining guidance on chlamydia screening
- reviewing patient notes to determine whether others have reported symptoms related to chlamydial infection

- developing a practice policy for chlamydia screening, treatment and referral

Needs assessment for chlamydia screening

The need for chlamydia screening can be established by reviewing practice data, epidemiological data and comparing the two.

The ***practice-defined approach:*** practice data can be reviewed to determine:

- the number of women and men who are screened for chlamydia
- reasons for offering screening
- proportion of positive tests by age and risk factor (under 25, multiple partners, unprotected sex as indicated by request for emergency contraception or pregnancy testing)

The ***epidemiological approach:*** the incidence and prevalence of Chlamydia can be monitored by reviewing the:

- number of men and women receiving screening from the general practice
- number of men and women receiving screening from another provider
- proportion of patients who test positive for chlamydia on samples that have been submitted by the practice
- proportion of positive sexually transmitted infection (STI) tests on men who were not tested through the local general practice

The ***comparative approach:*** practice data can be compared with community data to determine the:

- prevalence of chlamydia by age and risk factor in the samples submitted by general practices, GUM, family planning, and other clinical services

Clinical audit of chlamydia screening

Practice data and epidemiological data can be used to identify situations in the practice when chlamydia screening should be offered. Once standards and targets have been set, the proportion that are eligible for screening and those who are offered it can be audited annually. Variations in practice can be identifed and reasons for the variations can be discussed by the practice team.

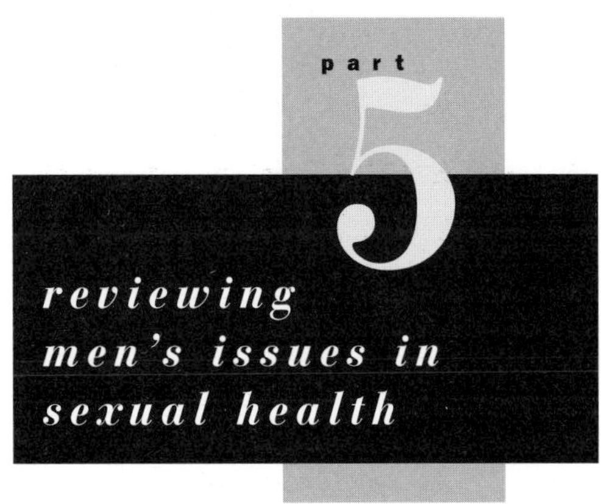

Needs assessment: assessing expressed and unexpressed need

General practice services are typically under-utilised by men. The assumption is often made that, since men don't use services, they are not in need of them. This may not be the case. As a first step in ensuring quality services for men, the practice should consider conducting an assessment of both expressed need – needs which are reflected through direct requests for services – and unexpressed need. This can be done in several ways:

The ***practice-defined approach:*** practice data can be reviewed to determine information on the needs of men who use practice services:

- proportion of men who have visited the practice within the last year
- proportion of men who have visited the practice for sexual health services
- types of sexual health services needed/requested
  - contraception
  - screening for STIs
  - preconception advice

The ***comparative approach:*** practice data can be compared with community data to determine the:

- proportion of male visits at other local practices
- proportion of men who receive sexual health services outside the practice
- types of sexual health services requested at other settings

This kind of analysis identifies the unique needs of the practice population in comparison with other local populations.

The ***epidemiological approach:*** the incidence and prevalence of STIs can be monitored by reviewing the:

- number of men requesting STI screening from the general practice
- number of men requesting STI screening from another provider
- proportion of male patients who test positive for an STI on samples that have been submitted by the practice
- proportion of positive STI tests on men who were not tested through the local general practice

The ***patient-defined approach:*** men's perceptions of their sexual health needs can be obtained via surveys and focus groups. These can be done both within and outside the practice. Assessments conducted within the practice will only obtain the views of service users; those conducted outside the practice can obtain useful information from patients who may not use practice services regularly, or who do not routinely express their needs. Outside assessments can be done through:

- health visitors, pharmacists, and other professionals who may be well placed to obtain information on men's health needs
- 'indigenous' interviewers – local men who live and work in the community in non-health settings such as leisure facilities, pubs or sports events
- researchers who may already be conducting local research/needs assessments on sexual health
- local statutory and voluntary organisations who may be willing to include questions about primary care needs on more general surveys that are being conducted

Mapping the community

Ask the men to draw a map of their local community. Then ask them to mark the places where they can go for information and services on sexual health.

On a second sheet of paper, ask them to write down all the places that they have identified. For each place, list the barriers to getting information and services. For each barrier that has been identified, ask the men to make suggestions for removing it. Bring this information back to the practice team for review and discussion about implementing the proposed solutions.

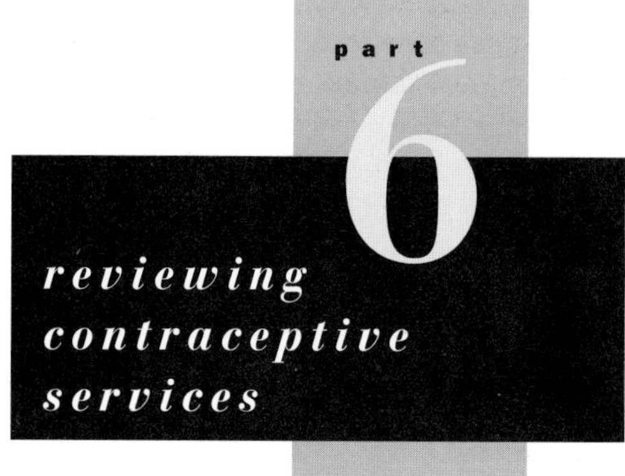

part 6 reviewing contraceptive services

Critical incident analysis: problems with oral contraception

example

A patient suffers a blood clot whilst taking oral contraception.
A patient becomes pregnant whilst using oral contraception.

An analysis of these incidents would involve relevant members of the PHCT in:

- discussing the factors which might have been involved in causing the event
- reviewing variations in counselling and prescribing
- considering the frequency of review, to ensure that patients are taking the pill correctly and know what to do should they have a stomach upset, forget to take a pill, or are prescribed an enzyme inducing drug
- reviewing the patient's case notes to establish whether care should be changed in the future to prevent such an occurrence
- identifying courses of action which might prevent it happening again in the future

- seeking out clinical guidance on prescribing and counselling protocols for oral contraception and reporting this back to the group
- developing a practice policy or a simple checklist to guide practice in the future

Clinical audit: prescribing combined oral contraception

The following checklist is based on the standards outlined in Chapter 6. This checklist can be used to review those patients on the practice list who are already prescribed combined oral contraception, document variations in clinical practice, and monitor achievement of future standards.

COC prescribing checklist[5]

The conditions associated with unacceptable risk are:

- pregnancy
- breast-feeding, less than 6 weeks postpartum
- blood pressure greater than 160/100mm Hg
- arterial disease, including ischaemic heart disease and stroke
- deep venous, or other definite, thrombosis, or known high risk of this condition
- complicated valvular heart disease, significant atrial or ventricular septal defect
- severe recurrent migraine headaches, including those with focal neurological symptoms
- current breast, gynaecological or liver cancer
- active hepatitis
- severe (decompensated) liver cirrhosis
- major surgery with prolonged immobilisation, surgery to legs, prolonged immobilisation after fractures (temporary risk)

Needs assessment: assessing potential contraceptive needs

example

The practice wishes to establish the size of its target population for contraception and the prevalence of contraceptive use amongst the female target population.

1 Define the target population (for example women/men aged 15 to 44)
2 Review practice register to determine the size of these populations
3 Determine the number of women using contraception over the course of one year by reviewing patient records or prescribing records or item of service payment records (NB. Prescribing records will not include use of condoms as main contraceptive method.)
4 Record contraceptive use once for patients who have repeat prescriptions or changed prescriptions within the year

$$\frac{\text{Number of women aged 15 to 44 using contraception}}{\text{Number of women aged 15 to 44}} = \text{prevalence of contraceptive use in women}$$

When interpreting the data, it should be remembered that:

- the accuracy of the calculation will depend upon accuracy of patient records and practice register but will give some idea of size of target population and prevalence of contraceptive use
- contraception can be obtained from a number of sources and therefore the prevalence recorded within the practice population may be an underestimate of actual prevalence of contraceptive use
- contraceptive prevalence does not equal consistent or accurate use of contraception. People can discontinue methods without telling the practice.

Needs assessment: providing a choice of contraceptive methods

The ***practice-defined approach:*** practice data can be reviewed to determine:

- the proportion of women who have expressed dissatisfaction with their contraceptive method
- the types of contraceptives needed/requested

- the proportion of women who changed contraceptives within the last year
- the proportion of women who discontinued contraceptives within the last year

The ***comparative approach:*** practice data can be compared with community data to determine:

- the types of contraceptives offered at other practices and community clinics
- the uptake of different types of contraceptives in other settings
- the proportion of women in the practice post code area who are obtaining contraception elsewhere
- the types of contraception that are obtained from other settings

The ***epidemiological approach:*** practice data can be reviewed to determine:

- the number of unintended pregnancies that occurred as a result of reported contraceptive discontinuation
- the number of unplanned pregnancies that occurred as a result of reported switching to another method

The ***patient-defined approach:*** patients' preferences can be discussed via surveys and focus groups. These can be done both within and outside of the practice. Assessments within the practice will only obtain the views of service users; those outside the practice can obtain useful information from patients who may not use practice services regularly, or who do not routinely express their needs. Outside assessments can be done through health visitors, maternity services, TOP services, pharmacists, and other professionals who may be well placed to obtain information on women's contraceptive needs.

Clinical audit: reviewing contraceptive choice

Reasons for non-provision of particular methods can be reviewed by organising a discussion group with all relevant members of the PHCT. The discussion can be facilitated through a 'spider' diagram:

1 Draw or write the method to be discussed, in the middle of a large sheet of paper.
2 Supply each member of the PHCT with a pen.

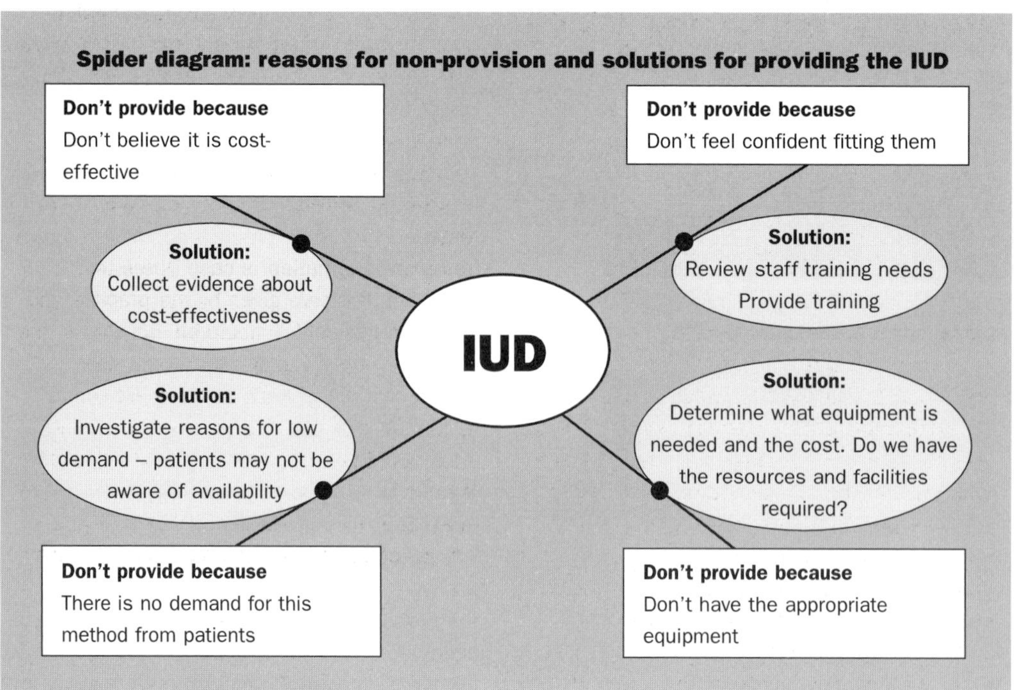

3 Brainstorm the reasons for non-provision of this particular form of contraception (the normal rules of brainstorming apply, ie each team member to make a contribution (unless they can't think of any reasons!), no judgements on/or discussion of suggestions until after they are all written down).
4 Each team member making a suggestion should draw a line coming from the method of contraception in the centre of the page. At the end of the line, write the reason for not providing this method.
5 After reasons have been exhausted, discuss each reason for not providing the method to establish whether it is something that can be overcome or something that really warrants not proving the method. Put solutions/course of action in boxes on corresponding line (as previous page).

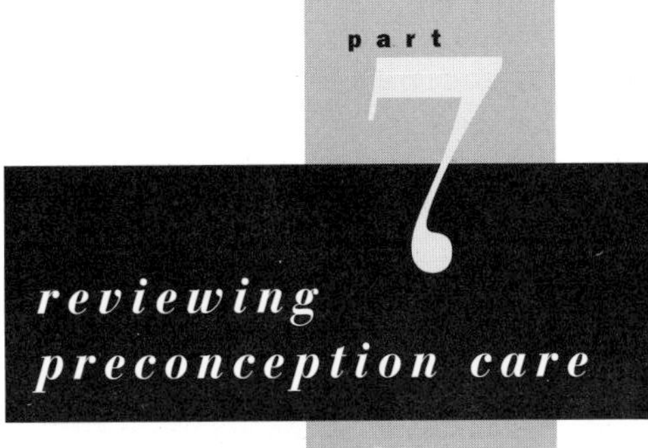

Preconception care includes programmes or services that are offered before or around the time of conception that improve the outcome of the pregnancy.

Needs assessment: access to preconception care

People can be surveyed to determine whether they are comfortable accessing sexual health services at family planning clinics and general practices. Raising awareness helps to ensure that more people will access services before they need them. This can be done opportunistically at the practice, by asking people who are attending for any type of health care whether they are aware of places that provide sexual health information and services.

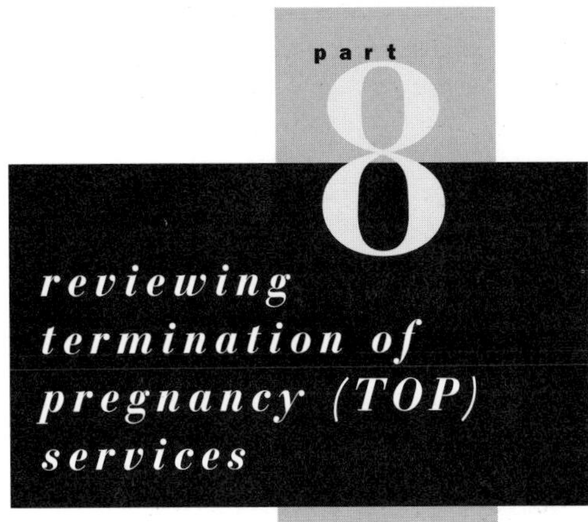

Critical incident analysis: emergency contraception failure

example

A young girl presents to the practice with an unplanned pregnancy and attributes it to failure of emergency contraception.

An analysis of this incident would involve relevant members of the PHCT in group discussion to brainstorm the factors which might have been involved in causing the event, and those courses of action which might prevent it happening again in the future. They may wish to look at variations in clinical practice amongst members of the PHCT with regard to the prescription of emergency contraception, and the reasons for these variations. Analysis of this event may also entail:

- reviewing the patient's case notes to establish the care given by the practice and whether it should or could be changed in the future to prevent such an occurrence
- a member of the PHCT seeking out clinical guidance on the prescription of emergency contraception and reporting this back to the group
- the PHCT developing a practice policy or a simple checklist to guide practice in the future.

Critical incident analysis: patient is refused a TOP referral

example

A complaint has been received from a patient that they have been refused referral for a TOP by a member of the practice.

It should be recognised that some critical incidents may be largely out of the control of the PHCT, for example the patient making the complaint may have been refused a termination of pregnancy because the pregnancy was beyond 24 weeks' gestation. Conversely, she may have been refused a termination because the particular doctor she saw had a moral objection to TOP. In both instances it is worth investigating the incident to establish whether there are any factors which could be influenced by the PHCT.

Late presentation for termination of pregnancy may warrant the PHCT reviewing its policy on health education/promotion, and taking measures such as putting up a poster in the waiting room stressing the importance of early presentation of pregnancy. The PHCT may also decide that it is worth liaising with the local school to address the issue through sex education.

The scenario where a doctor has a moral objection to TOP may result in the practice reviewing its policy on referring to other doctors within the practice.

Needs assessment: information needs about TOP services

Because the number of terminations occurring in individual practice populations is relatively low it is often inappropriate to adopt a comparative approach to data analysis. It is not normally statistically viable to make comparisons between incidence in the practice population and incidence in the local district unless data is aggregated over many years. For this reason a patient defined approach to needs assessment may be more appropriate:

example

The practice wishes to establish the information needs of the target population within its practice (women aged 15-44) with regard to its termination of pregnancy services.

The PHCT may wish to answer a range of questions including the following:

- What is the awareness level amongst the target population (15–44) of the availability of pregnancy testing at the practice?
- What is the awareness level of the availability of referral for termination of pregnancy and the need for early presentation?
- What do patients feel they need to know about what the practice offers?
- What do they feel they would need to know if they had an unplanned pregnancy?

A postal questionnaire could be designed and targeted at a sample of 15-44 year olds to address this issue. The information gathered could be used to shape health education/promotion strategies within the practice with regard to termination of pregnancy.

Needs assessment: accessibility of TOP services

example

The practice wishes to establish the accessibility of the termination of pregnancy service offered by the practice, from the viewpoint of the target practice population.

Structured interviews using largely open questions could be carried out with both users and non-users of this service to establish how accessibility could be improved. Questions which might be asked include:

- How would you feel about discussing an unplanned pregnancy with your family doctor
- What are your feelings about termination of pregnancy?

Depending on answer to above:

- How would you feel about asking your doctor for a termination?
- Is there anything that would put you off asking your doctor for a termination?
- Is there anything that would make it easier for you to ask your doctor for a termination?

Clinical audit: timeliness of TOP services

SELECT TOPIC FOR AUDIT

As with needs assessment the decision to review a particular aspect of care may arise out of a critical incident such as a patient being denied a termination as a result of the delay experienced in general practice.

topic

The practice wishes to audit the time taken between the patient's first presentation at the practice, requesting termination of pregnancy, and the date of their outpatient appointment.

PATHWAY OF CARE FOR TOP

The pathway of care experienced by the patient on requesting a termination of pregnancy may include some or all of the following stages. It should be noted that the time taken between Stages 4 and 5 and between Stages 5 and 6 is largely out of control of the general practice.

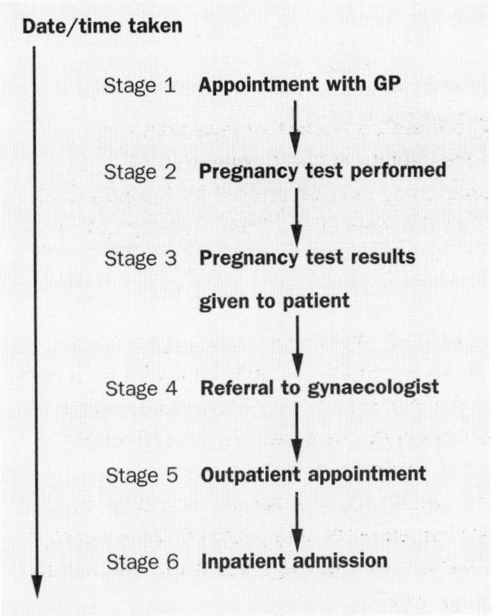

Date/time taken

Stage 1 **Appointment with GP**

↓

Stage 2 **Pregnancy test performed**

↓

Stage 3 **Pregnancy test results given to patient**

↓

Stage 4 **Referral to gynaecologist**

↓

Stage 5 **Outpatient appointment**

↓

Stage 6 **Inpatient admission**

SETTING STANDARDS

Since nationally recognised standards do not exist with regard to the timing of the above stages within general practice, it is necessary for the PHCT and perhaps the patient liaison group to reach a consensus based standard which is both appropriate for patients and achievable for staff. However guidance is available from the Birth Control Trust[6].

OBSERVING PRACTICE

Data can be collected retrospectively by reviewing the case notes of patients requesting termination of pregnancy to identify the length of time between each stage of the pathway of care. If case notes are not sufficiently detailed, then a prospective audit can be performed. It may be necessary to review case notes over a relatively long period because of the small number of termination requests made to a single general practice in an average year.

COMPARING PRACTICE WITH STANDARDS

If standards are not being met or there is variation amongst practice doctors then the PHCT should consider the extent to which the following factors influence the timing of the pathway of care:

- ease of obtaining appointment with GP: a prospective review of those requiring termination of pregnancy could be conducted to identify problems experienced by patients in obtaining an appointment. This may be particularly pertinent if one or more practice doctors have moral objections to termination of pregnancy
- need for pregnancy test: the practice may wish to establish what proportion of the pregnancy tests provided are in fact necessary, given that women may attend to request a TOP after having carried out a pregnancy test in their home or having a positive test from a family planning clinic. In such circumstances the provision of another test in general practice may add unnecessary delay to the pathway of care
- on-site versus laboratory pregnancy testing: if

the practice sends samples away for testing they may wish to review how long the test result takes to come back

- mode of referral: are there differences between doctors in terms of the way they refer to Gynaecology? for example by referring by letter, fax or phone, may result in significant variation in the overall time period between referral and outpatient appointment.

Service evaluation: multidisciplinary evaluation of timeliness of TOP services

example

The practice wishes to engage in multidisciplinary service evaluation of the timeliness of termination of pregnancy services.

After reviewing the timeliness of TOPs, the PCHT may find that there are areas where practice can be improved in both primary and secondary care.

Evaluation of the process will involve working with secondary care to review each step of the pathway of care for TOP (see page 186).

Critical incident analysis: non attendance

example

Patient attends for treatment of an STI after having failed to attend the initial GP appointment.

The patient's reasons for adopting this course of action would be explored in the consultation. However it may also be worth investigating the incident on a wider scale involving other members of the PHCT. Has this happened before? Can a mechanism be set up whereby the practice monitors non-attendance? What is the practice policy should a patient fail to attend an appointment? Are there any steps which the PHCT can take which makes the patient more likely to attend their appointment?

Needs assessment: incidence and prevalence of STIs

The overall incidence and prevalence of various STIs in the practice population can be established and compared with district level data by obtaining information from the following sources:

- practice data
- GUM data on referrals made by the individual practice
- district level data from KC60 forms submitted by GUM (available via health authorities)

As with TOP, the incidence of certain STIs may be sufficiently low to prevent meaningful comparison with district-level data except where data is available for several years.

Clinical audit: patient notification of STI test results

example

The practice wishes to review its mechanism for notifying patients of STI test results

There is no specific evidence on the most effective ways to inform patients of test results, an audit of this area will involve the PHCT in reaching a consensus about how to communicate test results. Many issues will need to be taken into account, including the maintenance of confidentiality, the promptness of the notification system and ensuring that no-one is missed. Once a policy is set up this will allow PHCT members to compare their current practice with the standards they have laid down and to change areas of their current working which do not match the standards required. It is important to recognise that local standards and targets should be reviewed after the audit has run for a while to ensure that they are appropriate, achievable and relevant to clinical practice.

Service evaluation: referrals to GUM

example

The practice wishes to evaluate the efficiency of the referral system to GUM

After auditing their procedures for notifying patients of STI results, the practice may find that:

- patients with an STI are not always referred to GUM
- patients who are referred to GUM do not attend for treatment

The practice may wish to collaborate with GUM in establishing:

- the number of DNAs
- characteristics of DNAs (age, sex,etc)
- reasons for non-attendance or late attendance

The quality of sexual health services in general practice can be maintained by ensuring that services are:

- **appropriate for individual patient situations**
- **responsive to individual and population-based needs**
- **based on local and national evidence whenever possible**
- **co-ordinated with other primary, community and secondary care sexual health services**

The examples of good practice found in this book can be compared to your current practice, using a variety of methods. Methods for reviewing practice include critical incident analysis, needs assessment, clinical audit, and service evaluation.

Different methods are used in different situations, as follows:

- **Critical incident analysis is useful for reviewing individual patient situations and determining whether problems are isolated incidents or indicative of wider practice issues**
- **Needs assessment is helpful in determining whether current practice is responsive to patient, practice and population needs**
- **Clinical audit is used when there is local or national evidence of best practice. This evidence is used to establish standards which can be used to assess the quality of clinical care**
- **Service evaluation can be conducted when general practice services are part of a local sexual health strategy, or when general practices have specific sexual health interventions or objectives which are in need of assessment**

- ***Evaluating the effectiveness of contraception services for teenagers: audit methodologies***
  National Co-ordinating Unit for Clinical Audit in Family Planning (in press)

- ***Medical audit in general practice***
  Marinker M
  BMJ Publishing Group, 1995

- 'Managing change in general practice: introduction'
  Pringle M
  British Medical Journal, 304, 1992, 1357-58

1 ***Needs assessment in general practice,*** Gillam SJ and Murray SA, Royal College of General Practitioners, Occasional Paper 73

2 ***Promoting clinical effectiveness: a framework for action in and through the NHS,*** NHS Executive, Department of Health, 1996

3 ***Evaluation fundamentals: guiding health programs, research and policy,*** Fink A, Sage Publications, 1993

4 Priority appointment request card, Schering Health Care Ltd, Burgess Hill, West Sussex

5 see Chapter 6 of this handbook, 'Providing high quality contraceptive services in primary care' Guillebaud J and Hannaford P, 83-108

6 ***A model specification for abortion services,*** Paintin D, Birth Control Trust, 1995

Acknowledgements

We would like to thank all the clinicians we have worked with through the National Co-ordinating Unit for Clinical Audit in Family Planning and the Yorkshire Clinical Audit Unit, for providing examples of their work in audit and evaluation.

We would particularly like to thank Dr Kate Guthrie, (Consultant in Sexual and Reproductive Health Care, The Princess Royal Hospital, Kingston upon Hull), for providing us with information about her work in the multidisciplinary audit of termination of pregnancy services.

Janet Harris and Andrea Jones

useful organisations

This list is reproduced from the *FPA Contraceptive Handbook* (2nd edition, FPA 1997)

Abortion

Birth Control Trust
16 Mortimer Street
London W1N 7RD
tel 0171 580 9360

Cancer organisations

BACUP (British Association of Cancer United Patients)
3 Bath Place
Rivington Street
London EC2A 3JR
tel 0171 613 2121

Women's Nationwide Cancer Control Campaign (WNCCC)
Suna House
128-130 Curtain Road
London EC2 3AR
tel 0171 729 2229

Breast Cancer Care
Kiln House
210 New Kings Road
London SW6 4NZ
tel 0171 384 2344

Clinical guidelines and audit

National Co-ordinating Unit for Clinical Audit in Family Planning (NCU)
University of Hull
Hull HU6 7RX
tel 01482 466051

Clinical Outcomes Group (COG)
Quarry House
Quarry Hill
Leeds LS2 7UE
tel 0113 2545972

UK Cochrane Centre
Summertown Pavillion
Middleway
Oxford OX2 7LG
tel 01865 516 300

Disability

Spinal Injuries Association
76 St James Lane
London N10 3DA
tel 0181 444 2121

SPOD (Association to Aid the Sexual and Personal Relationships of People with Disability)
286 Camden Road
London N7 OBJ
tel 0171 607 8851

Family planning organisations

Faculty of Family Planning and Reproductive Health Care (FFPRHC) of the RCOG
27 Sussex Place
Regent's Park
London NW1 4RG
tel 0171 723 3175

Family Planning Association
2-12 Pentonville Road
London N1 9FP
tel 0171 837 5432
Contraceptive Education Service Helpline
tel 0171 837 4044

FPA Cymru
Grace Phillips House
4 Museum Place
Cardiff CF1 3BG
tel 01222 342766

FPA Northern Ireland
113 University Street
Belfast BT7 1HP
tel 01232 325488

FPA Scotland
Unit 10
Firhill Business Centre
76 Firhill Road
Glasgow G20 7BA
tel 0141 576 5088

FP Sales Limited
Unit 9
Ledgers Close
Nuffield Industrial Centre
Littlemore
Oxford OX4 5JS
tel 01865 749333

Margaret Pyke Centre
73 Charlotte Street
London W1P 1LB
tel 0171 530 3600

National Association of Nurses for Contraception and Sexual Health (NANCSH)
c/o EMY Secretarial Services
181 Kings Acre Road
Hereford HR4 OSP
tel 01432 344000

NI Association of Family Planning Nurses
86 Ravenhill Park Road
Belfast BT6 ODG

RCN Family Planning Forum
Royal College of Nursing
20 Cavendish Square
London W1M 9AE
tel 0171 409 3333

Scottish Society of Family Planning Nurses (SSFPN)
9 William Place
Scone
Perth PH2 6TF
Scotland

General women's health

Women's Health
52 Featherstone Street
London EC1Y 8RT
tel 0171 251 6580

Health promotion agencies of the UK

Health Education Authority
Trevelyan House
30 Great Peter Street
London SW1 2HW
tel 0171 222 5300

Health Education Board for Scotland
Woodburn House
Canaan Lane
Edinburgh EH10 4SF
tel 0131 447 8044

Health Promotion Agency for Northern Ireland
23 Hampton Park
Belfast BT7 3JW
tel 01232 644811

Health Promotion Wales
Ffynnon-las
Ty Glas Avenue
Llanishen, Cardiff CF4 5DZ
tel 01222 752222

Infertility

ISSUE (The National Fertility Association)
114 Lichfield Street
Walsall
West Midlands WS1 1SZ
tel 01922 722 888

CHILD
Charter House
43 St Leonard's Road
Bexhill-on-Sea
East Sussex TN40 1JA
tel 01424 732361

Human Fertilisation and Embryo Authority (HFEA)
Paxton House
30 Artillery Lane
London E1 7LS
tel 0171 377 5077

International family planning organisations

International Planned Parenthood Federation (IPPF)
Regent's College
Inner Circle, Regent's Park
London NW1 4NS
tel 0171 487 7900

Irish FPA
Unity Building
16-17 O'Connell Street
Dublin 1
tel 003531 8780366

Lesbian and gay support

Gay Switchboard
BM Switchboard
London WC1N 3XX
tel 0171 837 7324

Friends and Families of Lesbians and Gays
PO Box 153
Manchester M60 1LP

Medical organisations

British Medical Association
BMA House
Tavistock Square
London WC1H 9JP
tel 0171 387 4499

Committee on Safety of Medicines/
Medicines Control Agency
Market Towers
1 Nine Elms Lane
London SW8 5NQ
tel 0171 273 0289

Royal College of General Practitioners
14 Princes Gate
London SW7 1PU
tel 0171 581 3232

Royal College of General Practitioners (RCGP)
– Manchester Research Unit
Parkway House
Palatine Road
Manchester M22 4DB
tel 0161 945 6788

Royal College of Nursing
20 Cavendish Square
London W1M 9AE
tel 0171 409 3333

Menopause support

Women's Health Concern
PO Box 1629
London W8 6AU
tel 0171 938 3932

The British Menopause Society
(for professionals)
36 West Street
Marlow
Buckinghamshire SO7 2NB
tel 01628 890199

The Amarant Centre (private)
Churchill Clinic
80 Lambeth Road
London SE1 7PW
tel 0171 401 3855

National Osteoporosis Society
PO Box 10
Radstock
Bath BA3 3YB
tel 01761 432472

Natural family planning organisations

Fertility Awareness and Natural Family
Planning Service of Marriage Care
Clitherow House
1 Blythe Mews
Blythe Road
London W14 0NW
tel 0171 371 1341

Older people's sexual health

Age Concern
Astrol House
1268 London Road
London SW16 4ER
tel 0181 679 8000

One-parent families

National Council for One Parent Families
255 Kentish Town Road
London NW5 2LX
tel 0171 267 1361

Pharmaceutical organisations

Royal Pharmaceutical Society of Great Britain
1 Lambeth High Street
London SE1 7JN
tel 0171 735 9141

National Pharmaceutical Association
38-42 St Peter's Street
St Albans
Hertfordshire AL1 3NP
tel 01727 832161

PMS support

PREMSOC
PO Box 102
London SE1 7ES

National Association for PMS (NAPS)
PO Box 72
Sevenoaks
Kent TN13 1QX
tel 01732 741709

Pregnancy organisations

Maternity Alliance
5th Floor
45 Beech Street
London EC2P 2LX
tel 0171 588 8582

National Childbirth Trust
Alexandra House
Oldham Terrace
London W3 6NH
tel 0181 992 8637

Miscarriage Association
Clayton Hospital
Northgate, Wakefield
West Yorkshire WF1 8JS
tel 01924 200799

Stillbirth and Neonatal Death Society (SANDS)
28 Portland Place
London W1N 3DE
tel 0171 436 5881

Support after Termination for Fetal Abnormality (SATFA)
73 Charlotte Street
London W1P 1LB
tel 0171 631 0285

Psychosexual problems

Institute of Psychosexual Medicine
11 Chandos Street
London W1M 9DE
tel 0171 580 0631

Association of Sexual and Marital Therapists
Box 62
Sheffield S10 3TS

Relationships

RELATE - England
Herbert Gray College
Little Church Street
Rugby
Warwickshire CV21 3AP
tel 01788 573241
For local centres see telephone or local help directory

RELATE – NI
76 Dublin Road
Belfast BT2 7HP
tel 01232 323454

Marriage Counselling Scotland
105 Hanover Street
Edinburgh
EH2 1DJ
tel 0131 225 5006

Jewish Marriage Council
23 Ravenshurst Avenue
London NW4 4EE
tel 0181 203 6311

Marriage Care (previously Catholic Marriage Advisory Centre)
Clitherow House
1 Blythe Mews
Blythe Road
London W14 0NW
tel 0171 371 1341

Catholic Marriage Advisory Centre - NI
76 Lisburn Road
Belfast BT9 6AF
tel 01232 491919

Sex education

FPA
(see FPA, page 192)

Sex Education Forum
National Children's Bureau
8 Wakley Street
London EC1V 7QE
tel 0171 843 6000

Sexual health organisation (for professionals)

Society for the Advancement of Sexual Health (SASH)
PO Box 17
Cheltenham GL54 2YU
tel 01451 822551

Sexuality issues

The Albany Trust
The Art of Health & Yoga Centre
280 Balham High Road
London SW17 7AL
tel 0181 767 1827

Beaumont Society (information for transexuals and transvestites)
BM Box 308 G
London WC1N 3XX

Gender Dysphoria Trust
tel 01323 970230

STIs including HIV/AIDS

For details about NHS genitourinary medicine (GUM) services, contact the FPA Contraceptive Education Service helpline,
on tel 0171 837 4044
(Monday to Friday, 9am to 7pm)

National AIDS Trust
New City Cloisters
188-196 Old Street
London EC1V 9FR
tel 0171 814 6767

National AIDS Helpline
tel 0800 567123 (24 hour freephone)

Terrence Higgins Trust
BM AIDS
London WC1N 3XX
tel 0171 242 1010 (helpline)
tel 0171 831 0330 (administration)

Training (in family planning for doctors and nurses)

Faculty of Family Planning and Reproductive Health Care
27 Sussex Place
Regent's Park
London NW1 4RG
tel 0171 723 3894

English National Board for Nursing, Midwifery and Health Visiting
Victory House
170 Tottenham Court Road
London W1P 0HA
tel 0171 388 3131

Welsh National Board for Nursing, Midwifery and Health Visiting
Floor 13
Pearl Assurance House
Grey Friars Road
Cardiff CF1 3AG
tel 01222 395535

National Board for Nursing, Midwifery and Health Visiting for Scotland
22 Queen Street
Edinburgh EH2 1NT
tel 0131 226 7371

National Board for Nursing, Midwifery and Health Visiting for Northern Ireland
Centre House
79 Chichester Street
Belfast BT1 4JE
tel 01232 238152

Association of Nurse Prescribing
4 Crinan Street
London N1 9SQ
tel 0171 843 4517

Unplanned pregnancy

British Pregnancy Advisory Service (BPAS)
Austy Manor
Wootton Warren, Solihull
West Midlands B95 6BX
tel 0345 304030 for information

Marie Stopes House
108 Whitfield Street
London W1P 6BE
tel 0171 388 0662
tel 0800 716390 for information
on local centres

Young people

Brook Advisory Centres
(Head Office)
165 Gray's Inn Road
London WC1X 8UD
tel 0171 713 9000

Youth Access
1a Taylor's Yard
67 Alderbrook Road
London SW12 8AD
tel 0181 772 990

authors' and editors' details

eneral
and
he is a
don, and
.
of the
s
ctive
et Pyke
Centre, London.

Philip Hannaford MD, MRCGP, MFFP, DCH, DRCOG is Grampian Health Board Professor of Primary Care. He is former Director of the RCGP Manchester Research Unit.

Janet Harris BA, MA is Director of Health Care and Health Sciences, Department of Continuing Education, University of Oxford. She is former Deputy Director of the Department of Public Health Medicine, University of Hull.

Jaki Hunt DRCOG, MRCGP, MFFP was a general practitioner until 1991 and now works in sexual health (genitourinary medicine, pyschosexual medicine and family planning) and as an audit facilitator in primary care. She is national audit lead for the Institute of Psychosexual Medicine.

David Jewell MA, MRCGP is Consultant Senior Lecturer in Primary Health Care, University of Bristol, and a general practitioner in North Bristol.

Andrea Jones BSc, MSc is Project Officer at the National Co-ordinating Unit for Clinical Audit in Family Planning, University of Hull.

Louis Levy BSc, MSc, PhD, MIBiol, CBiol is Sexual Health Promotion Team Leader at *Health First*, the health promotion unit for Lambeth, Southwark and Lewisham, London. He specialises in training and development related to HIV and sexual health.

Trefor Lloyd has been involved in developing work with men for 15 years. He co-founded *Working with Men* and *the B Team* in 1985 and has written and spoken extensively on issues affecting men.

Philippa Matthews MRCGP, B Med Sci, DRCOG is GP Principal at Colston Health Centre in Birmingham. She also works for the Primary Care and HIV Project, Birmingham Health Authority.

Catti Moss MBBS, MRCGP is a general practitioner in rural Northamptonshire. She is a GP trainer and teaches medical students. She is also Medical Vice Chair of the RCGP Patients' Liason Group.

Theresa Nash BSc, RGN, Higher Dip HV, SN cert, FP cert is Senior Lecturer in Health Promotion and Primary Care (Sexual Health), Kingston University and St George's Medical School. She was previously Primary Care Sexual Health Facilitator for Bexley and Greenwich Health Authority.

Catherine Paterson MBBS, MRCOG, MFFP is Consultant in Community Gynaecology and Reproductive Health Care, St Mary's Hospital, London. She also runs a District Pregnancy Advisory Clinic, which provides counselling and termination of pregnancy services. She is a trustee of the British Pregnancy Advisory Service.

Yvonne Stedman MB, BS, MFFP, MRCGP, DGUM, DRCOG is Consultant in Family Planning and Reproductive Health Care and Honorary Lecturer at the Department of Obstetrics and Gynaecology, Birmingham University.

Gill Wakley MB, ChB, MFFP, MIPM is a general practitioner in North Staffordshire and Lecturer in Primary Care, Keele University. She is Examiner for the Membership of the Institute of Psychosexual Medicine and Accredited Leader in training for psychosexual medicine.

Joan Walsh BSc is Health Policy and Research Officer at the Family Planning Association and has wide experience of working in reproductive health care. She has recently been involved in the *It takes two* project run by the FPA/HEA Contraceptive Education Service, promoting contraceptive health care for men and women in a GUM setting.

Anne Weyman BSc(Soc), FCA is Chief Executive of the Family Planning Association. She is the Founder and Honorary President of the Sex Education Forum.